# 'Are You Afraid of Snakes?'

# A Doctor's Exploration of Alternative Medicine



C. Scott Mahan, MD

MedMaster, Inc., Miami

ISBN13# 978-1-935660-26-2
ISBN10# 1-935660-26-6

*Made in the United States of America*

Published by
MedMaster, Inc
P.O. Box 640028
Miami, FL 33164

## Acknowledgements

I extend a special thank you to my family and friends who have put up with my antics for the past five years. My three boys, Connor, David, and Thayer, are undoubtedly relieved that they will receive a break from my embarrassing stories. My wife and soulmate, Beth, tirelessly edited multiple iterations of my book and also allowed me to expose our personal life within the pages. I also thank my sister, Amy Tamargo, who read and reread my book despite practicing law and juggling the demands of a family. Also, I'd like to give a shout-out to my sister-in-law Jamie Mahan who provided proofreading and guidance, and also to my artistic brother-in-law David Kim, who along with his girlfriend Molly, produced the book cover. Dr. Stephen Goldberg, the head of MedMaster publishing, was willing to take a risk and publish a book outside the typical genre of his publishing house. He also provided excellent editorial support. Last, I thank the many "alternative" practitioners who poked and prodded me in an attempt to cure my many maladies. I have attempted to keep their identities anonymous, but Asheville is a small town so I am sure some will put two and two together. Nevertheless, I was always treated with compassion – no exceptions.

## Contents

# Preface

I spent the past five years exploring the wilds of alternative medicine. What is alternative medicine you might ask? How does it differ from complementary medicine? *Alternative medicine* refers to a non-mainstream practice used in place of conventional medicine, while *complementary medicine* is a non-mainstream practice used in conjunction with conventional medicine. Many disciplines, such as acupuncture, commonly fall into both categories. In researching this book, I have personally experienced approaches that are often at odds with my training as an infectious diseases specialist. My explorations opened my eyes to many different approaches to health and wellness. I have had my nasal cavity probed, my spine stretched, and my body bathed in crystal energy. My goal in writing this book is to take the reader behind the closed doors of alternative medicine to find out what really happens.

As a Western-trained doctor, I often hear my colleagues disparage alternative medicine, but most of their opinions are based on innuendo rather than a true examination of alternative practices. In researching this book, I visited each alternative practitioner with an open mind and a willingness to follow the prescribed recommendations. In relating my experiences, I hope to both entertain and educate. In an attempt to limit my bias for or against any particular practice, I approached each visit as a non-medical person might.

Prior to each experience, I read about the discipline on the practitioner's website. I also read about each discipline in *Alternative Medicine – The Definitive Guide*, which is written by alternative proponents and therefore presents each discipline from the perspective of a believer rather than a skeptic.[1] I then spent the next month or so doing my best to follow the advice given, and I reported on whether the malady for which I sought care has gotten better. Throughout, I described my experiences and the results in real time. Basically, I performed a trial of one – scientific method at its worst.

Only when I have completed the experience do I then subject the discipline to the scrutiny my evidence-based, Western training taught me. I ask if the purported basis for the discipline is plausible or if it is just a bunch of mumbo jumbo. I also research the basis and evidence supporting each discipline with the help of the published literature, which I then summarize at the end of each chapter. The last five years have been a lot of fun, at times painful, but always insightful. I look forward to having you join me on my exploration of alternative medicine.

Despite my use of *Alternative Medicine – The Definitive Guide* as my guidebook, you should recognize that information obtained from this source is not gospel. It clearly trumpets the perceived benefits of alternative therapies rather than evaluating the pros and cons. Despite its drawbacks, it was the largest and most complete compendium on alternative medicine at our local bookstore, and it effectively served to provide background to the theories and proposed benefits of several alternative disciplines. If interested in the other side of the argument, I refer you to the following books: *Trick or Treatment: The Undeniable Facts about Alternative Medicine* by Edzard Ernst and Simon Singh; and *Snake Oil Science: The Truth about Complementary and*

*Alternative Medicine* by R. Barker Bausell. For Internet sites that continually update current information about alternative medicine, I suggest *Science-Based Medicine blog, The SkepDoc* by Harriet Hall, MD; *New York's Memorial Sloan Kettering Cancer Center's herbal/botanical database;* and *The Cochrane Summaries*, all of which can be found with a simple Google search.

## Endnote

1 Trivieri, L., & Anderson, J.W. *Alternative medicine—the definitive guide* (2nd ed.). Ten Speed Press. 2002.

# Introduction

My eyes track the chiropractor as he circles my prone body. I try to stay relaxed, much as an antelope relaxes while a lion lurks in the tall grass. Finally, he grasps my head between his brawny arms and gives my neck a high-intensity crack. I gasp. My next instinct is to wiggle my fingers and toes to make sure I have not become a quadriplegic. Relief ebbs through me—my bodily functions are intact. How did I, a Western-trained doctor and self-proclaimed skeptic of all things "alternative," end up in this position?

In July 2009, the Centers for Disease Control reported Americans spend over $34 billion annually on "alternative medicines."[1] The amount spent on visits to chiropractors, acupuncturists, homeopaths, and other "alternative" practitioners, and on the medicines they recommend, is beginning to rival the out-of-pocket costs spent on traditional Western (modern) medicine. Parents are opting not to have their children vaccinated against lethal childhood diseases due to concerns of mercury toxicity, Guillain-Barre syndrome, and autism. I even have an acquaintance diagnosed with HIV who considered taking herbal remedies instead of his doctor-prescribed anti-viral medications. As a long-time disciple of Western medicine, I am forced to ask myself . . . What is going on? Has everyone gone crazy?

I practiced as an internal medicine doctor in the small town of North Wilkesboro, North Carolina, for several years. I had, and still have, several standard lines I say to my patients who inquire about the benefits of taking supplemental doses of various vitamins and herbal remedies. Included among these is: "If it really works, it likely would be proven." I then recite that the National Institute of Health now has a National Center for Complementary and Alternative Medicine, which funds research on alternative therapy. Therefore, if a well-designed trial had been conducted proving a therapy's benefits, we would know about it. It often appears the makers of these "alternative" or "natural" drugs have a vested interest in not doing these studies, which are likely to disprove the touted benefits of their remedies. If the patient is still listening to me, I usually go on to list examples such as vitamin E, which the medical establishment almost unanimously believed decreased the risk of heart attack and stroke. Almost all cardiologists recommended vitamin E to their patients 10-12 years ago, and to do otherwise bordered on malpractice. Subsequent studies found that vitamin E did not decrease the risk of heart attack or stroke and actually increased the risk of heart failure. Finally, I add, "Unless there is a well-proven benefit, why spend your money on something that is as likely to harm you as help you?"

By now, you recognize me for the skeptic I am. I have devoted my entire career to learning the scientific method. I believe in the necessity of well-designed, randomized, controlled studies to guide medical practices. But even I recognize the groundswell of enthusiasm for another way. Alas, modern medicine is largely to blame. The pressure to address patients' needs in 15-minute visits, prescribe an expensive medicine for every malady, and the lack of physical contact permeating current medical practice is undeniable. Alternative medicine presents a different paradigm, where the practitioner actually takes the time to listen to patients and helps them design a holistic treatment plan to achieve well-being.

In response to the growing fascination with alternative medicine, I have chosen to place my cynicism on the back shelf and undertake a true examination of its methods. I have an ambitious plan. For the next few years, I will place my health in the hands of alternative medicine practitioners. I will swallow every pill and suffer any embarrassment in hopes of finding the true path to well-being. I will chronicle my experiences, both good and bad, and form an opinion, subjective as it may be, to the underlying value of each method. First, let me outline my current beliefs, or some might say "misconceptions," about various alternative medicine practices. Despite my skepticism, I am not totally blind to the potential benefits of the "other way." I willingly refer my patients to chiropractors for lower back pain, I dabble in yoga, and I love a good massage as much as the next fellow. I place practices such as yoga, low calorie diets, stretching, exercise, meditation, and massage in my "I believe it works" category. My "maybe it works" category includes chiropractor care for lower back pain, acupuncture, hypnotism, vitamin C, zinc, and echinacea. My "you must be kidding" category includes copper bracelets, magnet therapy, homeopathy, reflexology, and others.

My internal medicine training in Portland, Oregon, followed by several years of practice in rural North Carolina really piqued my interest in "alternative medicine." Portland has a reputation (deservedly so) of being populated by progressive "granola" types. (I mean no slander here, as my wife, whom I met in Portland, clearly fits this billing.) In my medical practice in Portland, I was repeatedly surprised by the strange concoctions and fringe medical treatments patients tried. These ranged from herbal remedies I couldn't pronounce, to the practice of "cupping," where cups with suction are applied to the skin to mobilize blood flow and promote healing. After I relocated to rural North Carolina, I was inundated with a whole new spectrum of "alternative meds." Patients brought in bizarre concoctions passed down for generations, often made in the very "moonshine still" their grandparents had used. As an evidence-based,

Western-trained physician, I was very skeptical of these alternative therapies, some of which I felt bordered on dangerous.

I likely would have kept my opinions to myself had my wife not stirred me to action. She was reading a book by Dr. Andrew Weil, who emphasizes the value of testimonials. We are taught from day one of medical school to beware of testimonials. There is always the possibility of spontaneous cure, placebo effect, misdiagnosis, or excited endorphins, which may lead patients to mistakenly attribute their "cure" to a treatment that, when examined more closely, is without merit. One testimonial describes an unnamed doctor who "feels" cerebral impulses between the cranial bones. Needless to say, my cerebral impulses sounded an alarm! Of course, I was worried my wife would be brainwashed and turn to the dark side (she already had shown some tendencies). In that moment, I decided I would embark on a journey of enlightenment to decide for myself what works and what does not. I would use my scientifically trained brain and form an informed opinion regarding the merits of various alternative therapies. What follows is my quest for the truth about alternative medicine.

## Endnote


1 Nahin, R.L., Barnes, P.M., Stussman, B.J., et al. Costs of complementary and alternative medicine (CAM) and frequency of visits to CAM practioners: United States, 2007. *National Health Statistics Reports; no 18*. National Center for Health Statistics, 2009.

# Chapter 1 My Early Exposure to "Alternative Medicine"

I am 43. Up until this point, my life has gone pretty much according to script. I grew up in Gainesville, Florida, a small college town. I did my undergraduate work at Duke University in Durham, North Carolina, where I was "pre-med" like the majority of Duke students. I graduated from medical school at the University of South Florida in Tampa in 1993, and I was accepted into Internal Medicine residency in Portland, Oregon, at Oregon Health Sciences University. My grandfathers were doctors, my dad is a doctor, I have an uncle who is a doctor, and several doctor cousins. Suffice to say, I was not breaking any new ground. Conversations around the family dinner table were spiked with medical doctrine. My friends grew accustomed to the graphic medical discussions and barely batted an eye when they came over during our viewing of a home video of one of my dad's patients giving birth. (This was in the early 1980s, before it became customary for births to be filmed and posted directly onto YouTube.)

It was during my three years of residency and one year of chief residency in Portland that I was first confronted with "alternative medicine" as an accepted therapeutic option. The "left coasters," as we easterners call California, Oregon, and Washington inhabitants, seemed to have more interest in alternatives to standard "Western" practices. In the internal medicine clinic and on the general hospital wards, I was forced to investigate the potential interactions and side effects of non-prescription, alternative meds. Ginkgo biloba, ginseng, saw palmetto, and St. John's wort were all the rage. Not to mention the Asian patients who brought in Chinese herbal remedies, the ingredients of which went largely undiscovered. I became acutely aware that a whole lot more "doctoring" was going on than I had been exposed to in my books during medical school.

My schooling in "non-Western" medicine continued during an 8-month stint in Ghana, Africa. I have had a fascination with Africa stemming from a childhood in which I was entranced by weekly episodes of Mutual of Omaha's *Wild Kingdom* hosted by Marlin Perkins. This interest was further sparked during residency when I was introduced to tropical medicine—malaria, tuberculosis, and leishmaniasis. How exotic! During chief residency, I spent my spare hours plotting a way to spend time in Africa prior to starting a real job. Like many Americans, I am geographically challenged. While trying to arrange a position in Uganda, I accidentally signed up for a volunteer position in Ghana. As you may know, Uganda is situated in Eastern Africa near the famed wildlife reserves often seen on *Wild Kingdom*, while Ghana is far to the west. Western Africa is more noted for the crush of humanity than the call of the wildebeest. Fortunately, my geographical incompetence led to one of the best experiences of my life.

I arranged a posting as a volunteer doctor in Pramkese. Pramkese is a small village of a few thousand persons in the south central region of Ghana – a temperate, previously heavily forested region, just six degrees off the equator. After convincing my fiancée, Beth, to join me on the adventure, I began planning in earnest. I assembled my own library of medical texts on tropical medicine, pediatrics, obstetrics, and basic surgical techniques. I learned how to prepare my own microscope slides to diagnose malaria. I beefed up my tropical medicine knowledge. My dad even gave me last-second instructions on how to perform an emergency cesarean section! (Basically, throw some Betadine on the mother's abdomen, cut with scalpel, extract baby, and call for help.)

My time in Ghana exceeded my expectations. Although we did not have elephants or lions in our backyard, we were embraced by the community and became intertwined in everyday village life in a manner I would not have thought possible for a foreigner. Beth and I spent eight months in Pramkese. I worked in a small government health clinic, and Beth, a lawyer by training, taught English to elementary students in the village school. I never had to perform that emergency cesarean section, but I was introduced to several new forms of alternative medicine.

At times, I felt I had been placed in a time machine and transported back 100 years to the pre-antibiotic era in the United States. While I diligently attempted to cure the ills of the villagers with my small armamentarium of antibiotics and Western therapies, the general populace continued to seek "alternative" remedies. Even my medical staff was not immune. One day, a street peddler drove into town with a loudspeaker on the top of his pickup truck. He was selling a "cure-all tonic" that purportedly healed piles (hemorrhoids), back pain, fevers, malaise, headaches, and more. To my astonishment, villagers I didn't even know existed emerged from the woodwork to place old bottles, cans, and plastic jugs in the bed of the peddler's pickup truck to be filled with a dark brown concoction. I could not help but roll my eyes and give a look of dismay when my chief medical officer, Mary, who had trained in Germany, brought forward her own bottle to be filled. It would have been convenient to attribute the behavior of the villagers to poverty and the overwhelming expense of going to see me at the Community Health Clinic, but I knew otherwise. It was well known it cost only $0.25 to be seen by "the doctor," and even this nominal fee would be waived if necessary.

While in Ghana, I cared for several patients who came to me for a second opinion after traditional remedies had failed. One gentleman came to the clinic and complained of chronic pain in his right ear. He had tried several herbal remedies recommended by a local practitioner, but he was not getting better. With my otoscope in hand, I peered into his ear canal. To my surprise, his ear was jammed full of crushed herbs! After I briefly irrigated his ear with some warm water, he was miraculously cured. This case and similar ones did little to bolster my faith in traditional healing methods. I was aware, however, that I only saw the failures rather than the potential masses of persons who claimed to have been cured by Ghanaian traditional healing.

Villagers also sought care from the local Juju priestess, Akosua Manu, who was rated as just “okay” according to Kwasi, one of our close friends. He said she was a relatively weak Juju practitioner compared to the Juju priests in the neighboring villages. Women frequently sought the priestess’ assistance with the pains of labor and other maladies. In general, my interactions with her were limited. The exception was when Beth and I made a special trip to her home and place of practice, to formally meet her and get a better idea of what she was about. Kwasi, acting as our translator and guide, had arranged the meeting. We brought the recommended bottle of peppermint schnapps as an offering, and we were invited into the back of her house. Akosua seemed quite amicable as she sat in the back of her small clay house with a corrugated steel roof. At the front of the room was a stool for her to sit on and a makeshift shrine littered with several partially or fully emptied schnapps bottles. She guided us to some wooden planks serving as benches near the shrine. Then she sat down on the stool inches in front of us and began answering our questions while exchanging the required pleasantries. Beth and I both tested our rudimentary knowledge of the local dialect, Twi. Mid-conversation, she appeared to disengage. She fell into a trance and developed a distant gaze in her eyes. She then threw white powder over her face and at us while we sat uncomfortably close to her. She began thrashing around with a machete while babbling unintelligible words. At this point, Kwasi leaned in and discretely informed us she was now possessed (not a striking revelation!). After a while, she calmed down, took a swig from one of the schnapps bottles, and returned to sanity. At this point, we nervously stood up and prepared to leave. She quickly jumped up and asked to have her picture taken with us. She also suggested we proclaim our allegiance to one another at the next village gathering. I gave a tentative nod to this suggestion, and we made a hasty retreat.

I was reluctant to publicly condone Akosua's practices to the village. My skepticism of her practices was based on my brief interaction with her at her home, and also having seen at least one case of negligence on her part. A few weeks prior, I had cared for a 14-year-old girl who was near comatose due to meningitis. The child had only been brought to me after having failed to respond to the ministrations of the Juju priestess. I don't know what Juju therapy entailed, but apparently antibiotics were not part of the prescription. Needless to say I was not eager to endorse her methods. Fortunately, I managed to sidestep the whole ethical dilemma of supporting her practices via a public proclamation, and we managed to remain on good terms. She may not have been the most powerful Juju priestess, but I decided I would rather not take a chance of her spreading any bad juju in my direction. Although my time in Ghana was among the best of my life, after eight months of third world medicine, I was ready to return to the United States.

I accepted a job as a general internist in North Wilkesboro, North Carolina, the proclaimed birthplace of NASCAR.

North Wilkesboro and adjacent Wilkesboro are basically one town located in the foothills of the Appalachians with a combined population of just over 7,000 persons. I anticipated that now that I was away from the "granola" crowd of Portland, Oregon, and the tribal traditions of Ghana, I would no longer be exposed to alternative medicine. Boy, was I wrong! The Wilkesboros opened up a whole new window to my thinking about "alternative" medicine. Now I got to experience "Appalachian" medicine.

My first encounter with "Appalachian" medicine came as the result of the passing of a much-loved elderly general practitioner in town, Dr. Jack Dawson. Since I was a new practitioner in town and one of the few doctors accepting new patients, several of Jack's patients joined my practice. As a result, I became familiar with several concoctions he had dreamed up that the local pharmacy happily compounded for his patients. Depending on a patient's perceived malady, be it coughing with congestion, stomach upset, or nervousness, he or she could order up the appropriate "Dawson's mixture." I could literally write a prescription for Dawson's mixture #1, #2, or #3 based on a person's complaints, and the pharmacy would provide the corresponding concoction. Believe it or not, I could even write a prescription for "snake oil," another brew that Dr. Dawson had created and was highest in demand. To this day, I can't help but chuckle when I think of Jack Dawson dreaming up a mixture and naming it "snake oil," a name that has been used to belittle numerous "cure-all tonics" that have been peddled over the centuries with claims to fix all maladies (not unlike those tonics being sold by the traveling vendors in present-day Ghana). Jack clearly had a sense of humor, and for the most part, his concoctions were relatively benign combinations of already available over-the-counter medications, such as liquid diphenhydramine (the ingredient in Benadryl), milk of magnesia, and liquid acetaminophen (Tylenol), occasionally mixed with some stiffer substances such as belladonna or codeine. They appeared to cause no harm, and the patients definitely imbued these concoctions with special healing powers that went above and beyond any of the individual ingredients.

Aside from Dr. Dawson's concoctions, I remember an elderly woman I admitted to the hospital with pneumonia. She was 92 years old and came into the emergency room clutching her own bottle of cough syrup brought from home. She swore her cough syrup was much superior to the ones she might receive in the hospital. It turned out her cough syrup was actually Robitussin mixed with "white lightning" (another name for moonshine and a testament to the surviving illegal distilleries that still abound in the region). I figured that she had made it past 90 years old, so who was I to deprive her of this apparently effective and calming remedy?

Another woman came to me from a local chiropractor and informed me she had hepatitis (inflammation of the liver). I asked her to explain the basis for this concern, as I could not detect any of the telltale signs of liver problems, such as jaundice (yellowing of the skin), nausea, or abdominal pain. She said her chiropractor had made this diagnosis and had sent her to me to have blood drawn to confirm the diagnosis. Needless to say, the tests all came back normal, and I became somewhat wary of this chiropractor. I have always maintained that chiropractors should focus on skeletal problems rather than stray outside their area of expertise.

On a regular basis, I was introduced to folk remedies and local superstitions that were remarkable in their ingenuity. My interest in these "alternative" therapies made me susceptible to the occasional prank. One of my patients who had "come down from the hills" caught me off guard. He noticed I was suffering from a cold with a runny nose. He pulled two buckeye nuts out of his pocket and told me that if I rubbed them on whatever "ailed" me, it would improve. I dutifully rubbed the nuts over my nose and sinuses. He then informed me he was sure I would be feeling better soon because he had used the very same nuts this morning on his hemorrhoids and was now free of pain!

After six years in the Wilkesboros, I uprooted my growing family: my wife, Beth; two sons, Connor and David; and a female dog named Jack. I accepted a three-year position to specialize in infectious diseases at Case Western University in Cleveland, Ohio. Over the next three years, I trained in a highly specialized field of medicine and practiced in advanced medical centers. My interest in alternative medicine took a back seat to the scientific method and evidence-based Western medicine. I continued to observe with interest the public's fascination with echinacea, vitamin C, zinc, and other remedies to stave off colds and prevent disease despite a lack of studies showing definite benefit.

At the end of three years, I accepted a position at MetroHealth Medical Center in Cleveland. My primary role was to teach medical students and residents evidence-based medicine. My focus was on infectious diseases, HIV care, and running the county tuberculosis program.

You, the reader, are now just about caught up. I just celebrated my 43rd birthday, and I have finally gotten the gumption to start writing about my experiences. Although I can already reflect on my life to this point and see lots of accomplishments and adventures completed, I feel the creep of middle age. Will I ever get around to those big adventures I dream of . . . exploring the Amazon, hiking the Inca trail to Machu Picchu, visiting Australia and New Zealand, and returning with my whole family to West Africa? I feel the clock ticking, but I am unable (or unwilling) to go right now because of all the responsibilities of life – primarily my job and my family (another son, Thayer, was born in 2007). I wonder if I will be healthy enough to enjoy these adventures ten to fifteen years from now. Some mornings when I wake up, particularly after having played basketball the night before, I am not sure my body will hold up. It seems my list of chronic maladies grows by the day. With this in mind, I decided it was time to try something new (or should I say something "alternative"?).

Here is my plan. In a city teeming with world-class, modern medical facilities – the Cleveland Clinic, Case Western/University Hospitals, and the MetroHealth Medical Center – I plan on shunning all I hold true in favor of the dark side. Over the next few years, I will shed my cynicism and give "alternative medicine" a true chance. Equipped with an expansive guide to alternative medicine purchased by my wife at a local bookstore, I will see if my maladies can be healed. I plan on trying each new discipline of "alternative medicine" for at least a month and to record my experiences for posterity.

# Chapter 2 What Ails Me

Like many who have reached middle age, my list of complaints is long. Life goes by too fast to adequately address the multiple, nagging aches that cling to us over the years. Among my ever-growing list of ailments are headaches. I have suffered from frequent headaches since childhood. My first recollection of having one was during middle school while playing pee-wee football. The headaches became more frequent and severe during my residency. I was fortunate to rotate through a headache clinic as part of my internal medicine training. There, I diagnosed myself with a combination of tension and non-classical migraine headaches. As doctors are prone to do, I began treating myself . . . unsuccessfully. I had little relief with over-the-counter medications, such as Tylenol, ibuprofen, and Naprosyn. A friend prescribed me an antidepressant, amitriptyline, for headache prevention. It had little impact on my headaches, but I did sleep well while taking it, and it caused me to have a very dry mouth. Taking a mere 25 mg dose, only about one-fourth the dose I often prescribe to little old ladies, I was dead to the world. Normally a light sleeper, I could now sleep through a three-alarm fire. When I did awaken, I felt groggy until noon, which is not a good state for a busy, third-year medical resident. When the antidepressant failed to offer relief, I thought maybe poor vision was the cause of my headaches, so I made an appointment with an ophthalmologist, but my eyes were fine. I moved on to allergy meds, thinking maybe I had sinus allergies, all to no avail.

Fortunately, the frequency of my headaches usually wanes after a month or so and I forget about them for a while. This cycle changed a few years back when I was nearing the end of my infectious diseases fellowship. I developed daily crushing headaches centered behind my right eye. These headaches woke me from my sleep and were associated with nasal stuffiness and tearing in my eye. Aha! I had a new diagnosis . . . cluster headaches. At some point in the intervening years between childhood and fellowship, I started taking Maxalt, a potent prescription medicine, a few times a month for my headaches. Now I was taking it two to three times a day with minimal relief. Finally, I could stand it no longer, and I went to the emergency room seeking relief. I had a CT scan of my head, which was essentially normal, and my diagnosis of cluster headaches was confirmed. I spent six hours in the emergency room, and I was given no acute therapy for my headache. I merely received a referral to a neurologist and a prescription for prednisone and verapamil (both prescribed based on my suggestion to the ER doctor – they are thought to help cluster headaches). My unsatisfying experience in the emergency room led me to understand why people might seek alternatives to "modern" medicine.

I saw the neurologist a few weeks later. He added little to my therapy but extracted a $40 co-pay for his efforts. I half-heartedly took the prednisone and verapamil for the next few months and eventually tapered off these meds. Ultimately, my headaches returned to their normal pattern.

My other maladies include bilateral heel pain, diagnosed as plantar fasciitis by a podiatrist. After playing basketball, I hobble around for several days, walking like a gorilla on the outsides of my feet. I tried icing my feet, ibuprofen in mega-doses, rest, and every brand of over-the-counter orthotic insert available, all without relief. In desperation, I even allowed a baby-faced podiatry student to inject my heels with steroids, hoping for improvement. Finally, I resorted to pricey tailor-made orthotic inserts, which I have worn religiously for the past five years. According to the podiatrist, the inserts, made of hard plastic with a small amount of rubber cushioning over them based on a mold of my feet, are designed to keep my feet in the "neutral position." It sounds a bit hokey to me, but I have largely been able to return to my normal activities, with the exception of running. Despite the success of the orthotics, I still have an element of heel pain that persists, and I have basically ruled out ever walking barefoot again. Also, the inserts guarantee no shoe will truly feel comfortable again. Imagine buying a nice, cushioned pair of running shoes and then throwing a couple of rocks in them before placing them on your feet!

My third chronic complaint is my lower back. I know this is extremely common, largely because almost half my patients have the same complaint. My lower back is stiff in the morning and aches throughout the day. Having three young boys doesn't help. In fact, my backaches clearly worsen over the course of a long family vacation and improve when I return to work. I rarely have radiation of pain into my legs, but at times the back pain is quite limiting. I have resorted to stretching, something I despise. I pride myself on being the least limber person in the world. I don't think I have touched my toes since I was in utero. I live on anti-inflammatories. It is a wonder I haven't bled to death from stomach ulcers. I wear a back brace when I play basketball and sleep with a board under my mattress.

My fourth major concern is my memory, or lack thereof. I ruled out a career in politics early on when I realized I am abysmal at remembering names. For the life of me, I can't recall the plot line of most movies I have seen. Beth reassures me this is normal, but with increasing frequency, she has been bringing up that we should obtain long-term health care insurance. All of this would be a bit more humorous if my mother didn't currently reside in an Alzheimer's care facility, where she has been since the ripe old age of 67. In the hope of staving off dementia, I read anything I can find about Alzheimer's, and as a result I have cycled through daily ibuprofen, daily aspirin, vitamin E, and ginkgo biloba. But invariably, after taking anything for a while, I run across new research debunking the benefits and pointing out possible detrimental effects. Beth encourages me to do mind games to stay sharp, but I suck at crossword puzzles, get bored with Sudoku, and fall asleep when doing brain teasers. To make matters worse, when I had the head CT for my headaches, the resident who initially reviewed the CT noted some "mild" brain atrophy (shrinkage). Fortunately, the final report did not confirm this, but I admit I am too scared to look into it further. I, of course, assume the worst. I figure I have another 15-20 years before senility sets in.

Do I have any other medical concerns? I am ashamed to admit there are more. I suffer from periodic bouts of insomnia. My right shoulder appears to have some form of rotator cuff tendonitis that leads to soreness after activities such as basketball or throwing a ball. I periodically get pain in my left groin region after sporting activities. I have attributed this to a lower abdominal muscle strain, but its failure to fully improve after prolonged periods of inactivity has led me to a sneaking suspicion that it may instead be a hernia (basically my intestines protruding through a weakness in my lower abdominal wall). I repeatedly give myself a half-hearted physical exam to search for the telltale bulge of a hernia that is more obvious when coughing or bearing down. I can't clearly identify any such bulge, but as an internist, I remember missing a few small hernias in my patients that the surgeon picked up. A hernia? A true sign of old age!

Last, although not really a malady, I am overly fertile. My wife is reeling from the effects of three young boys, ages 10, 8, and 3. She is too stressed to reliably remember to take "the pill." Thus, she often refuses to be in a closed room at night with me for fear of becoming pregnant. She has of course requested I get "fixed." I do not feel I am broken; therefore, I have done my best to delay this inevitable procedure. Why delay, you may ask? I do not desire any more children, but I do have a reluctance to entrust "my boys" (and I don't mean Connor, David, or Thayer) to a surgeon. My friends reassure me that having the big "V" is really no big deal, but I know otherwise. I remember one patient I cared for in North Wilkesboro who developed an infection at the site of the vasectomy. The result was that he was hospitalized, and his scrotum was left open for daily dressing changes by young nurses while he received IV antibiotics. One exposure like this is enough to force any man to think twice before having a vasectomy. I suggested to Beth that we try herbal remedies to cure my sexual potency, but when I last checked, the door to our bedroom was still locked.

Now that I have chronicled my maladies in excruciating detail . . . here is my plan: First, I will make an appointment with an internal medicine doctor at my hospital for a full check-up. We will see how the "modern" medical experience goes. Thereafter, I will begin my exploration of the "dark side." I plan on systematically trying different "alternative" medical modalities for my various complaints. My sister Amy has brought up the point that if something works too well, then my journey in alternative medicines will come to a quick end, and I won't have any material for my planned book. This is a risk I am willing to take. I figure if the experiment goes too well and all my ailments are cured, then sacrificing writing a book is a small price to pay. I am fairly confident it will take a while to solve all my problems, and if they are resolved, I need only to play a few games of basketball to discover some new problems.

# Chapter 3 Checking Under the Hood – My Initial Check-up

In accordance with my plan, I make an appointment with a local internal medicine doctor for a check-up prior to experiencing the "alternatives." This will be a good way to confirm my self-diagnosed ailments and to see what modern medicine might have to offer, although I already have a pretty good idea after practicing general internal medicine myself for many years.

My first attempt at scheduling an appointment does not go well. Remember, this is in the very hospital where I work. I call the number listed online to schedule a medical visit. I am placed on hold for ten minutes. When I finally get to speak with a living, breathing person, she tells me I need to be transferred to the employee line. After ten more minutes on hold, I again speak with someone who says I have been misinformed and I, in fact, need to call back the first number. I am back where I started. I call the original number, and I am forced to wait ten more minutes before someone new finally picks up the phone. Now, the most incredible thing happens: I am told there are no available appointments in the next two weeks, and that visits can only be scheduled within the month they will occur, so I will need to call back. Finally, I hang up. My father, who spent his career attempting to improve healthcare in this country, would be appalled. He often expounds how medical clinics could use a good lesson from Disney with regard to customer service and crowd control. Where is Mickey Mouse when I need him?

Months pass before I can summon the will to again attempt to schedule an appointment. Truth be told, I am not a big fan of going to doctors, Western or otherwise. To top it off, my wife has noticed a growth on my scalp right in the middle of my growing bald spot. I have noticed this crusted area frequently breaks off when I am combing my hair, and it is prone to bleeding. Now I am forced to see both a medical doctor for a regular check-up and a dermatologist to diagnose the recurring growth on my scalp.

I call to schedule a dermatology appointment and, amazingly, I get through after only 15 minutes. I am scheduled to see a doctor the next day. Next, I again try to schedule a general medical appointment. Sadly, I once again go through a similar rigmarole as the first time, but after repeated attempts I finally get an appointment scheduled for a month down the line.

Finally, the day of my appointment with the internist arrives. I check in at the desk and take a seat in the crowded waiting room. Even as a doctor, I admit that crowded waiting rooms give me the willies. Does the man next to me have tuberculosis, maybe pertussis? After a while, one of the nurses notices me cowering in the corner with my hand covering my mouth. She sheepishly calls me back and apologizes that the doctor is running a bit behind. Knowing I too am a doctor, she allows me to bide my time working on one of the computers in the back of the clinic. Forty-five minutes later, I finally sit down with the doctor. The doctor sits at the computer and reviews my history and asks if I have any ongoing problems or concerns. I tell him about my headaches and insomnia. I decide not to mention my chronic lower back pain or other maladies as I don't want to be perceived as a hypochondriac. He has me sit on the exam table; he looks in my mouth, feels my neck, and listens to my heart and lungs with a stethoscope. He obviously does not think I look ill. Who can blame him? Compared to some of the patients in the waiting room, I must look like a picture of health. He seems to be going through the expected steps with little afterthought – perhaps checking off the required boxes on a list. He then refills my prescriptions for Maxalt, which I take for headaches, and Ambien to help me sleep. My blood pressure and weight are all okay. He recommends I have blood work done to check my lipids, and then he is out the door. We spent about 20 minutes together. This is a pretty long visit in my field. I know all too well the deficiencies of "modern" medicine. I invested several hours of my time for a rather uninformative visit, but I have the medications I want and a generally clean bill of health. I can understand why the average person might feel unfulfilled after a similar experience: very little hands-on attention and not much time with the doctor despite long waits and heavy costs. Enough of "Western" medicine . . . I am ready to see what "alternative" medicine can do for me.

# Chapter 4 Heal Thyself – Naturopathy and Homeopathy

Naturopathy focuses on the stimulation of one's "vital force" or one's own healing capacity. It comprises a holistic approach, which facilitates the body's natural mechanisms to be well. There is a focus on diet, exercise, and lifestyle changes aided by the use of dietary supplements and homeopathic remedies. The first components sound reasonable, but I have long been skeptical of homeopathy. I originally set my sights on seeing a dedicated homeopath, but I am unable to find anyone for whom homeopathy is the sole component of their practice. Instead, the homeopathic community in Cleveland is mostly comprised of medical doctors providing homeopathic remedies on the side to supplement their income. I find a licensed naturopath recommended by a close friend. Her website appears very professional and we have the common bond of both having received our training in Portland, Oregon – hers at the National College of Natural Medicine and mine at Oregon Health Sciences University.

The doctor's office is on the second floor of a historic building. There is no sign outside to indicate its presence. This is clearly a word-of-mouth establishment. The waiting room is small, and the smell of incense wafts through the air. On one wall are shelves displaying a vast array of available supplements and remedies, much like the display of hair care products that confronts you as you enter a beauty parlor. There is an inviting photo depicting an empty dock extending out on a tranquil mountain lake. On the side wall is a stand with various teas for consumption and purchase. While able to appreciate the calming feel of the place, I can also appreciate its money-making potential.

Two young women wait in line at the checkout counter. A third person, a meek gentleman, stands to the side in the waiting room. He waits patiently to purchase some supplements displayed on the shelves. Additionally, he makes a point of catching the attention of a visiting naturopath as she walks by in the hall to thank her for help with his "case." He then looks my way, and in a conspiratorial tone, informs me I will not be disappointed. Apparently, he recognizes me as a newbie based on the intake papers clutched in my hands. He gives me a knowing look – I am about to join their secret fraternity.

While waiting for my turn to check in, I grab a flyer that addresses flu vaccines. Being an infectious diseases doctor, I am extremely wary of any condemnation of vaccination. The flyer discourages people from getting vaccinated. It claims "vaccinations are not 100% safe because they carry altered forms of the offending pathogen (bacteria or virus) or secretions from the organisms." I am not happy about this statement despite its partial veracity. I am more concerned about the statement that flu vaccines "in fact, paralyze the immunity." This is untrue. The point of a vaccine is just the opposite. It stimulates the immune system, encouraging it to make more cells that recognize a potential pathogen, so that when the body is again exposed to that pathogen, it is able to respond with a more rapid and vigorous immune response and thereby prevent infection. The flyer goes on to recommend a homeopathic alternative called "Mucococcinum," which is a preparation of "two homeopathic bacterial fractions and one viral fraction." This concoction sounds disgusting. Is it someone else's mucus in a bottle? I think I will stick with vaccines for the time being.

After I wait only a few minutes, the doctor of naturopathy ushers me into her spacious office/exam room. I sit down on a love seat opposite her large wooden desk. On the far side of the room is a typical exam table. Shelves filled with homeopathic and medical books cover the walls. I recognize a few internal medicine and obstetric texts gathering dust that appear to be over twenty years old. In contrast, closer to her desk are several folders and homeopathic reference books well-worn from frequent use. The doctor sits down behind her desk and flips open her laptop. Over the next hour and a half, we review the extensive questionnaire I completed prior to my visit. It covers my past medical history, current medical complaints, and lifestyle. She uses this questionnaire as a jumping off point for more detailed questions about each of my complaints. Throughout the entire visit, she diligently taps away on the keyboard and periodically refers to the folders and reference books at her disposal. Despite writing notes while we talk, she remains very warm and engaged during my visit.

In some ways, the visit reminds me of a typical visit to a general medical doctor. The biggest difference is the length of time she spends with me and the depth of the questions probing my history. The hospital that employs me would not tolerate me spending over an hour with each of my patients. She asks me about my headaches and tries to define their frequency, location, triggering and exacerbating factors. She asks about remedies I have tried in the past and the impact of my diet or sleep. She asks similar in-depth questions regarding all of my complaints. She shows a particular interest in my bowel regimen, the consistency and frequency of my stools, and whether I have any skin problems. She even delves into possible sources of angst stemming from my childhood. I try not to disclose how my best friend Craig and I tortured my little brother, John. Could repressed guilt from having John retrieve toys from hornet-ridden crevices really be the root of my headaches? We discuss my insomnia, lower back pain, chronic foot pain from plantar fasciitis, and my Type A personality. I am impressed. She is thorough and yet remains relaxed, in no rush at all.

After getting more and more specific with her questions, she leans back in her chair and contemplates my various maladies. Finally, she proclaims, "I think I know what is going on." I lean forward in my seat and wait for the answer with baited breath. After an extended pause, she says, "You have inflammation." The unifying diagnosis hangs in the air for a few seconds as we both contemplate its significance. I stifle a guffaw. After over one hour of probing questions, no stone has been left unturned, and this is the answer. Inflammation. I am incredulous. In my profession as an infectious diseases doctor, inflammation is a symptom rather than a diagnosis in its own right. I have no doubt I could declare inflammation to be the problem in all of my patients and be correct 99% of the time.

My naturopath is not done. The next part of my diagnosis is even more intriguing. She concludes my adrenal gland is out of whack. Apparently, my cortisol (a hormone produced by the adrenal glands) levels are not following the appropriate diurnal rhythms, hence my insomnia. She inquires if I would like to have my cortisol levels checked via a saliva test. I balk at the $151 cost, and we agree to proceed with empiric management and consider the test at a later date. Now that we have a diagnosis, she goes to work developing a treatment regimen.

First, she suggests some exercises I should do for my back and feet. She places two tennis balls in a sock and demonstrates how to use these to massage my lower back and neck using the floor or a wall as resistance. She suggests some stretching exercises for my feet and recommends I pick up marbles with my toes to strengthen my foot muscles. Also, I should hang upside down from my hip crease to create a gap between my vertebrae and to focus on building my "core" muscles. These all seem like reasonable suggestions, exercises one might learn from a physical therapist.

Only when she starts to devise a regimen of dietary supplements and homeopathic medications does she really surprise me. She seems vexed while trying to find the appropriate remedy for my headaches. She pores over one of her books on homeopathic remedies, struggling to find the correct treatment. It appears my headaches do not fit into any of the well-categorized groups outlined in her text. She probes deeper, asking me about the location of my headaches: "Are they more on the right or the left side? What triggers your headaches? What time of day do your headaches occur?" Finally she pauses and looks up from the book laid out in front of her. "You might think this next question is a bit odd." She does not disappoint. She asks, "Are you afraid of snakes?" Am I mishearing her? No, she actually asked if I am afraid of snakes! The implication is this fear might have some bearing on the chosen headache remedy. "No," I state. "I actually am quite fascinated by snakes. In fact, we own a ball python named Monty." Disappointed, she again immerses herself in her text. After flipping through a few more pages, she inquires if being hungry precipitates my headaches. Happily, I say, "Why yes, I often get a headache when I am hungry or I miss a meal. In fact, I am often able to stave off a smoldering headache by getting something to eat." She seems pleased with this information and adds two homeopathic medicines to the regimen, Nux Vomica and Tuberculinum. Not the prettiest-sounding medications, but I hold my tongue.

The doctor prints out my personalized treatment plan. The focus is on an "anti-inflammatory diet," several exercises, dietary supplements, and four homeopathic medications. She explains that homeopathy is founded on the "law of similars." Basically, the goal is to administer a substance that provokes the very symptom you are trying to cure, but at very miniscule doses. "In fact," she explains, "the more dilute the dose, the more powerful the effect." As she expounds on this bedrock principle of homeopathy, I think to myself how very counter-intuitive and illogical it seems. Already I can tell I will not be benefiting from any "placebo effect" due to my inherent skepticism.

With two pages of printed out treatment plan in hand, the doctor personally checks me out and gives me the listed remedies. After two hours I have in hand eleven prescribed remedies to cure my "inflammation" and control my adrenal gland. I leave strangely satisfied. Despite being $400 poorer, I have received two hours of a doctor's personalized attention, and I have a dizzying array of new therapies to try out.

Soon after my visit to the naturopath, I realize that among the many remedies recommended, the biggest challenge will be adhering to the diet, or more specifically, the "anti-inflammatory diet." There are many vocal proponents of this and similar diets, both among naturopaths and the general public. In fact, as I drive to work a few days after my appointment, I tune into a short segment on National Public Radio interviewing Lisa Cimperman, a dietitian at University Hospitals in Cleveland, discussing the anti-inflammatory diet. The rationale behind the anti-inflammatory diet is that there is a direct link between the foods we eat and the amount of inflammation in our bodies. Certain foods, such as organic fruits and vegetables, are considered anti-inflammatory, whereas other foods, such as those that are heavily processed or high in saturated fats, are considered pro-inflammatory. According to Mrs. Cimperman, the evidence for these diets originates in studies that assessed life expectancy and health outcomes in large populations and then attempted to link these outcomes to the subjects' diets. Her conclusion was, although the findings are intriguing, there is no definitive evidence that a diet low in inflammatory foods is beneficial.

The guidelines for my "anti-inflammatory diet" are to eat more essential fatty acids (found in raw seeds and cold-pressed oils), bioflavonoids (found in organic vegetables and fruits), and foods high in vitamins C, E, B3, B6, biotin, copper, magnesium, selenium, and zinc. Foods to avoid include red meat (except grass-fed beef), processed oils, dairy, commercially processed eggs, pre-packaged foods, alcohol, coffee, and peanuts. As I read the list, I begin to cringe. This is not going to be easy. I live on dairy, alcohol, coffee, and nuts. Give up my morning java and my evening beer? What is the point of living if I can't enjoy myself? I recently read that coffee is the number one source of anti-oxidants in the American diet. And isn't a beer a day good for you?

As I read the diet out loud to Beth, a smirk spreads across her face. She is going to enjoy watching me suffer! We decide the first step will be to go to Whole Foods, our local organic food store, or "Whole Paycheck," as I like to call it. I despise this store. The fruits and veggies look great, but boy are they pricey! I don't see many persons using food stamps in here.

As I enter "Whole Paycheck," I immediately encounter rows upon rows of immaculate fruits and vegetables. I love strawberries, and the beautiful mounds of strawberries call to me. I notice there is one stack labeled "organic" strawberries and an identical mound next to it that are apparently conventional strawberries. They look exactly the same to me. In fact, the same company produces both the organic and conventional strawberries. The only noticeable difference is a small emblem identifying one set of packages as "organic." The berries all appear red, juicy, and delectable. I then notice the price difference. The organic strawberries are $4.69 per package and the non-organic $2.69. You must be kidding me. I begrudgingly grab a package of the more expensive, organic berries. I pick out a few organic vegetables (I am not a big veggie eater), some organic eggs, grass-fed hamburger meat, and some soy milk. My spirits hit a low point when I see the bill. The price is over $50 for a single sack of groceries.

I arrive home, look over my upcoming diet, and decide to indulge in one last night of decadence . . . beer, cheese, hamburger derived from a poorly treated cow, and maybe even some pre-packaged, highly processed baked goods. I tell myself, "Tomorrow, I begin the austerity . . . ahem, 'anti-inflammatory' diet."

As part of my therapeutic regimen, my naturopath prescribed seven supplements and four homeopathic remedies. The homeopathic remedies pique my interest the most. The goal of the medications, to the best of my understanding, is to decrease the inflammation in my body and regulate my adrenal glands, and in doing so, cure me of headaches and insomnia. Although I am inherently skeptical, I am eager to give them a try. After I get home, I lay out all the pills for my wife to admire. As I calculate the total number of remedies (10 pills, 10 drops, 2 scoops, 7 pellets, and 2 teaspoons) that I am supposed to take each day, I am overwhelmed. Will there be any room left in my stomach for that organic anti-inflammatory food I just purchased? Here is a rundown of the prescriptions and my understanding of their purposes:

1) Aller-C – A dietary supplement of quercetin, vitamin C, and bioflavinoids. According to the manufacturer, it is a "potent combination formula used to moderate the inflammatory response. Quercetin promotes decreased production of histamine, and the 60 citrus bioflavinoid complex supports the strength of capillaries." Interestingly, I have never heard of quercetin before, but when I Google it, I

am able to find circumstantial evidence for the manufacturer's claims. I am strangely reassured.

2) B-complex vitamin – Not much to say here. Even in the small village of Pramkese, Ghana, the villagers believed B-complex vitamins are imbued with magical healing powers.

3) Omega-3 Fish Oil capsules – Again, hard to argue with this one. Even the venerated source Wikipedia states fish oil capsules "are known to reduce inflammation throughout the body."

4) Vitamin C, calcium citrate, and magnesium citrate powder – Even after I read the product insert, I am not sure why I am taking this one. It appears to be primarily for bone health. It comes in a powder that when mixed with water, fizzes and tastes like Alka-Seltzer.

5) Seriphos (phosphorylated serine) – The bottle states it is an "adaptogen and adrenal support" agent. These are foreign terms to me. The manufacturer's website expands on the benefits of phosphorylated serine. It is purported to enhance memory and to impact circadian cortisol rhythms. The website excerpts a few random and very small studies as evidence for these claims. Mainly, it is selectively quoting the researchers who did the studies as justification for their claims; not very hard scientific evidence, but intriguing.

6) Linden Flower extract – All I can find about this one is it "promotes relaxation." This sounds good to me. Hopefully, it will have the same impact as my evening beer that has been unceremoniously eliminated in accordance with the "anti-inflammatory" diet!

7) Fruit anthocyanins – pure, concentrated syrup of grapes, blueberries, pomegranate, aronia berry, elderberry, and

raspberry. What are aronia berries? The website associates anthocyanins with many possible benefits, including anti-viral, anti-bacterial, anti-cancer, and basically anti-everything-bad properties.

These supplements cost a cool $150 for one month's supply. I realize I am now indistinguishable from several of my patients and from some of my wife's neurotic friends, who are frantically popping pills, going on periodic fasts, and getting "high colonics" in hopes of achieving natural health. Well, there is no turning back now.

Now we come to a class of remedies that in my mind are truly "alternative." Homeopathy has always intrigued and perplexed me. First, there is the "law of similars," whereby a remedy is selected to provoke the very symptoms one is trying to treat. This sounds a little bit like desensitizing someone to an allergen. One might imagine it works in a manner similar to a vaccine, which primes the immune system to develop a response to similar stimuli. Thus, it assists your natural immunity in responding to an inciting agent and decreases subsequent "inflammation."

The second premise of homeopathy is that increasingly dilute doses are increasingly potent. This is hard for me to stomach, and it throws a big wrench into my immune stimulation hypothesis. Both vaccinations and desensitization to allergies work on the principle that higher doses of the antigen (or substance to which one is allergic) provoke increasing immune responses. Basically, when an allergist desensitizes someone to an allergen (the substance to which they are allergic) he introduces the offending substance in sequentially higher doses. This is the opposite of homeopathy, which starts at slightly higher doses and sequentially decreases the dose with claims of increasing potency. I understand that when some homeopathic remedies have been tested in modern labs, no trace of the labeled ingredient can be found. My natural reaction is that this proves the medicine is a fake. The true believer sees otherwise and states that only the "essence" of the labeled ingredient remains, further substantiating the increasing power at greater dilution. Despite my skepticism, I understand that in Europe homeopathy is a mainstream medical therapy. What is behind Europe's fascination with homeopathy? Is it because it is less expensive than traditional medicine? Perhaps it reflects a stubborn support for a discipline with German roots. Homeopathy sounds well and good if one is treating a child with a cold, which will likely get better regardless of the treatment, but what if the child has a life-threatening illness, such as meningitis? With these thoughts in mind, here are the homeopathic remedies I have been prescribed and a bit of my research regarding their intended uses:

1) Lycopodium – It is derived from an evergreen plant in Europe and North America. It has been used since the Middle Ages for a broad spectrum of ailments ranging from gout to digestive disorders. It can be used for chronic insecurity, fear of an upcoming event, sleeplessness, nightmares, headaches, and more. I don't think I have any overwhelming insecurities, but I definitely fear my upcoming bouts of insomnia and headaches.

2) Tuberculinum – I find an incredibly long list of indications for this one. This medicine is intended for those with a family history of tuberculosis and/or for those prone to colds, allergies, or other respiratory disorders. To me, this is the oddest of the prescribed medications, especially since I oversee the county tuberculosis program. I'm having a hard time determining why this one was prescribed. The Internet provides an extremely long list of potential afflictions or traits that are benefited by taking this medication,

including the treatment of "incipient tuberculosis." As I peruse this long list of potential maladies cured by tuberculinum, the only one I see pertaining to me is "deep brain headaches."

3) Nux Vomica – This one sounds disgusting! According to Boericke's *Materia Medica* (originally published in 1927 but still used today), "Nux is preeminently the remedy for many of the conditions incident to modern life. The typical Nux Vomica patient is rather thin, spare, quick, active, nervous, and irritable. He does a good deal of mental work; has mental strains and leads a sedentary life, found in prolonged office work, overstudy, and close application to business, with its cares and anxieties." Following that description are about twenty pages of symptoms for which it might be useful, including lumbar back pain, insomnia, and headaches. Of all the medications so far, this sounds like the one for me.

4) Calcarea Carbonica – According to Boericke, its "chief action is centered on the vegetative sphere, impaired nutrition being the keynote of its action; the glands, skin and bone, being instrumental in the changes wrought. Again, it is good for incipient phthisis" (an archaic name for tuberculosis). As I read over these remedies and the cookbook-like fashion in which they can be prescribed, I can't get over the feeling this is similar to how medicine was practiced many, many years ago, during a time when people generally died at the age of 40. Among the 19 pages of symptoms that might be cured with Calcarea Carbonica, I find insomnia, back pain, and headaches listed. I'm feeling better already.

As I read over the descriptions of the many possible uses of these homeopathic remedies, I harken back to the time when medicine was practiced much differently. For direct comparison, I decide to pull out a few of my ancient medical texts. One such text, *The Principles and Practice of Medicine* by William Osler, MD, published in 1899, preaches that the best way to treat tuberculosis is to "make a patient grow fat" and place him or her in the open air. Diabetes can be treated with "opium" or, alternatively, with "valerian root." It seems traditional medicine has come a long way, but homeopathy remains unchanged.

Over the ensuing weeks I do my best to adhere to the complicated regimen of supplements. I make up a calendar so that I stay compliant with the prescribed dosages. It is kind of fun doling out a handful of pills each evening, none of which are too noxious. In addition to taking the pills, I am following the dietary recommendations. My wife certainly approves of the healthy dietary alternatives I have chosen.

Two weeks after starting the naturopath's recommended regimen of pills and the anti-inflammatory diet, I begin a busy rotation in the hospital. As if on schedule, my insomnia strikes. I faithfully take the prescribed remedies, but my inability to sleep is worse than ever. No sleep, combined with no morning coffee, is a brutal combination. I manage to survive a busy first day after no sleep without too much problem. On night number two, I go to bed tired but nervous. I wonder, "What if I can't sleep again?" As I lie down in bed, my heart starts to race. This is a bad sign. I strive to stay "natural." I want to give the naturopathy a chance. I check the clock every fifteen minutes, and around midnight I realize I am no closer to sleep but much closer to another sleep-deprived night. Just thinking of another sleepless night followed by a busy day at work makes my heart beat even faster. Finally, I break down and take an Ambien (a sleeping pill). This buys me 3 ½ hours of sleep. Not enough for someone who needs eight hours a night, but enough to allow me to survive day number 2 at work. I repeat this pattern the following two nights, attempting natural sleep followed by a brief Ambien-induced coma. I am a train wreck. I finally am forced to drink coffee in the morning just to survive the day.

On the fifth night, I decide it is time to try something different. I force myself to go for a pre-dinner run (more of a stumble in my sleep-deprived state); I stay up one hour later than usual; I read my book; and I convince my wife to "have relations" with me. I manage to sleep about five hours without the help of Ambien. Finally the cycle seems to be breaking.

On the sixth night, I play basketball in the evening. I am so tired that I have lost control of my limbs; I find myself uncontrollably fouling the man I am guarding. No one is mistaking me for Michael Jordan. That night, I repeat my new routine of staying up late, reading (it is getting hard to focus), and "having relations" with Beth. She really is very tolerant of me. My routine is rewarded with nine hours of blissful sleep. The following nights, I sleep well even without my wife's assistance. I have finally shed the brutal yoke of insomnia. It does not appear my Lycopodium, Nux Vomica, or Calcarea Carbonica, all of which claim to treat insomnia, helped in any way. Or perhaps the opposite is true, and they are responsible for my wonderful night of sleep – I just had to wait until enough time had passed to appreciate their benefits. Maybe . . . but I don't think so. It is easy to see how one might interpret the results to his own liking.

What about my other complaints? I have had a pretty good stretch regarding my headaches. During my week of insomnia, I have some minor headaches, but I never have to resort to taking my prescribed Maxalt. Since I began sleeping again, I have had no major headaches. My head might still get a little achy, but nothing disabling. Could this be a sign the Tuberculinum, Nux Vomica, and the Calcarea Carbonica are doing their intended job? Who knows? I suspect cutting back my coffee intake and the near elimination of alcohol are largely the reason. Maybe it is my more relaxed outlook, thanks to the Linden Flower extract.

My back, hip, and foot pains are unchanged. I suppose had I more rigorously adhered to the exercise and stretching program this might not be the case, but the anti-inflammatory diet clearly is not doing the trick. The multiple anti-inflammatory and "adrenal adaptogen" substances I have been taking are not making a difference either. I have continued with my regular exercise routine: biking to work (nine miles each way) one-two times/week; basketball one-two times/week; maybe a trip or two to the gym for some weight lifting and stretching; and chasing my kids around. After any of these activities, lifting and stretching aside, I feel pretty inflamed the next day. Perhaps the key to the anti-inflammatory diet's working is not exercising too vigorously. If so, I am afraid it might be a net negative for one's health.

After a little over a month of adhering to the naturopathic routine, I come to the following conclusions: I am very impressed with the amount of time the naturopathic doctor spent with me. This amount of time would be unheard of in a traditional medical practice. I think the lifestyle modifications, both dietary and exercise, prescribed by the naturopath are fairly common sense and similar to what a standard nutritionist and physical therapist might recommend. Some aspects of the "anti-inflammatory" diet are obvious, such as eating natural foods, adding more fruits and vegetables to your diet, and avoiding processed foods and saturated fats. Again, these are not groundbreaking principles. I am less sure about the restrictions on coffee and alcohol. The unique components of the naturopathic experience are the supplements and the homeopathic remedies. I can see the allure of these relatively inexpensive remedies. You can look up your symptoms in a reference book and then find any number of "natural" supplements and homeopathic remedies. This ability to determine your own treatment plan, with the naturopath's assistance, is very empowering. Unfortunately, beyond these admirable qualities, these remedies fall flat. If I am going to spend $150-$200 a month on remedies, I want to see some proof they work beyond what is written in a century-old book. I would like to think medical science has advanced the practice of medicine even just a little bit since Boericke wrote his homeopathic treatise, *Materia Medica*, in 1929. Just because it is written in a book does not make it true. Despite the many fallibilities of modern medicine, I believe there is a role for proof of principle. I admit my six weeks experimentation with Naturopathic medicine was just that – experimentation – but I certainly have my doubts, which have been magnified the more I have learned. I like the holistic approach to medicine, but I think my money would be better spent by seeing a nutritionist and a physical therapist (and it might even be covered by my health insurance).

## Naturopathy

**Cost of initial consultation:** $150-$350

**Cost of follow-up visits:** based on length of visit (15-minute visit – $30-$50; 1 hour visit – $100-$200)

**Cost of prescribed remedies:** $100-$300/month combined cost

**Covered by standard insurance policies:** No

**Published research:**

There are few rigorous studies in this field. There are three randomized clinical studies and one cost analysis, all conducted by the same group of researchers at the Canadian College of Naturopathic medicine.

1) The authors concluded that naturopathic care successfully lowered the risk of cardiovascular disease determined by a reduced Framingham 10-year cardiovascular risk score.[1] - Limitations of this study include the lack of a hard endpoint such as heart attack or stroke; instead choosing a reduced Framingham risk score to be a reliable indicator of benefit. Perhaps the results should not be surprising because the main intervention was promotion of healthy lifestyle and nutrition. It is impossible to separate out the possible benefit of the added naturopathic dietary supplementation.

2) In this study the authors concluded that naturopathic care reduced anxiety through a combination of counseling, deep breathing relaxation techniques, a daily multivitamin, and the herbal medicine, ashwagandha.[2] - Of note, both psychotherapy and naturopathic care led

to significant decreases in anxiety. Limitations of this study were that there were too many differing variables in treatment between the two groups. One is unable to conclude if the herbal remedy, dietary counseling, or lack of psychotherapy led to the measured outcomes.

3) The authors found that naturopathic care was beneficial for rotator cuff tendinitis as compared to doing standard physical therapy exercises alone. The naturopathic care group received dietary counseling, acupuncture, and an enzyme formula called Phylogenzym.[3] - The study format makes it impossible to determine what component of the naturopathic intervention led to the measured benefit – in this case a decrease in pain score. Was it the phylogenzym or the acupuncture?

4) A fourth study by the same group of Canadian researchers found naturopathic care was cost-effective as compared to standardized physiotherapy education for the treatment of chronic lower back pain.[4] - One should note that chronic lower back pain seems to respond to any intervention provided enough time is allowed to pass. The naturopathic group received exercises, dietary advice, and acupuncture, so it is hard to know which component, if any, led to the perceived benefit.

## Homeopathy

**Cost of initial consultation:** Varies widely depending on type of practitioner seen. Homeopathy is practiced on the side by a wide range of practitioners including naturopaths, MDs, chiropractors, and pharmacists.

**Cost of follow-up visits**: Varies based on type of practitioner.

**Cost of prescribed remedies:** $8-$30/remedy (available online, at natural food stores, and practitioners' offices)

**Covered by standard insurance policies:** No

**Published research:**

There is little evidence in the literature to support the use of homeopathy for any specific condition. In fact, many of the basic tenets of homeopathy are in direct opposition to established concepts of chemistry and physics.[5,6,7,8]

# Endnotes


1 Seely, D., et al. Naturopathic medicine for the prevention of cardiovascular disease: a randomized clinical trial. *CMAJ*, 2013;185(9): E409-E416.

2 Cooley, K., et al. Naturopathic care for anxiety: a randomized controlled trial ISRCTN78958974. *Plos One*, 2009;4(8):E6628-E6629.

3 Szczurko, O., et al. Naturopathic treatment of rotator cuff tendinitis among Canadian postal workers: a randomized controlled trial. *Arthritis and Rheumatism*, 2009;61(8), 1038-1045.

4 Herman, P.M., et al. Cost-effectiveness of naturopathic care for chronic low back pain. *Altern Ther Health Med.* 2008; 14(2): 32-9.

5 Altunc, U., et al. Homeopathy for childhood and adolescence ailments: systemic review of randomized clinical trials. *Mayo Clin Proc.*, 2007; 82(1):9-75.

6 Cucherat, M., et al. Evidence of clinical efficacy of homeopathy. A meta-analysis of clinical trials. HMRAG. Homeopathic Medicines Research Advisory Group. *Eur J Clin Pharmacol*, 2000; 56(1):27-33.

7 Shang, A., et al. Are the clinical effects of homeopathy placebo effects? Comparative study of placebo-controlled trials of homoeopathy and allopathy. *Lancet*, 2005;366(9487):726-32.

8 Jonas, W.B., et al. A critical overview of homeopathy. *Ann Intern Med.*, 2003;138(5): 393-9.

# Chapter 5 Oh, My Aching Back – Chiropractor

This past year, I joined my sister's church group on a mission trip to Nicaragua. I am not the religious type, but I do love an adventure, and the opportunity to travel to Central America with my sister was too good to pass up. Fortunately, I had not yet read *A Gringo Nightmare*, the tale of an American journalist falsely accused of murder in Nicaragua. This gentleman was left to wallow in a Nicaraguan jail as a frenzied populace called for his head. Somehow the lucky fellow managed to escape back to the United States.

Thankfully, my experiences were a bit more mundane. My role on the trip was to join one other doctor, a pediatrician, in providing basic medical care at a series of rural outreach clinics. My colleague had traveled to Nicaragua with the group before and would be handling the lion's share of the preparation. I just needed to show up and see patients. Rumor had it that the majority of patients we would see were not particularly sick. Despite this, we would be providing a valuable service as well as spreading goodwill. I also confirmed that religious conversion was not a requirement for receiving medical care – something to which I strongly object. There's nothing like being told to submit to the cross before you can be seen by the doctor.

You may be wondering where my back comes into this story. Each day while in Nicaragua, we would set off from our plush accommodations (basically men's and women's barracks) and travel to various makeshift clinics. Sometimes we set up shop in the spare room of an elementary school or church, and other times we relieved the doctors in busy government health clinics. The one constant in all this was we brought our own ergonomically challenged plastic chairs to sit in while seeing patients. I noticed over the course of the trip that my lower back got stiffer and stiffer. I resorted to lying on the floor between seeing patients to perform various yoga maneuvers such as "up dog" and "down dog." My contortions entertained the children to no end. Despite the subtle chuckles and outright finger-pointing at the "loco gringo doctor," I performed maneuvers that would make my yoga-loving wife proud.

The pain in my back was bearable until one of our last clinics. We traveled to a remote spot on the western coast. Rather than riding in our normal school bus or the air-conditioned Volkswagen camper, we traveled in the dreaded "Rhino Rally" (named after a similar-appearing vehicle at Busch Gardens, Tampa). An hour-long ride over unpaved, pot-holed dirt roads in the back of a large truck with no apparent shocks and no padded seating was enough to transition my back pain from an annoyance to true discomfort. Maybe I would have avoided true invalid status had I not foolishly agreed to play tennis with my sister at the hotel in the capital city of Managua, where we spent our last night before our departing flight home. Swinging a racquet and bending over for dead tennis balls on an unforgiving tile tennis court was the final straw.

Fortunately, my first week back at work was not overly busy, and I spent considerable time lying on my back on the floor of my office between seeing patients. After a week of little improvement, I decided it was time to see a chiropractor. Who is better qualified to treat back pain? Despite the fact that chiropractors are widely embraced, I have always viewed them through wary eyes. I value my spinal cord, and the thought of someone manipulating my vertebrae (which protectively encircle the spinal cord) scares me. I may seem like a hypocrite. I willingly refer my patients with lower back pain to chiropractors if the patient requests it, which they often do since the referral helps with insurance reimbursement. Despite making these referrals, I remain skeptical whether the patients, or I in this instance, will truly benefit.

According to my reference book on alternative medicine, chiropractic care is the second largest primary health care field in the world. The goal of the chiropractor is to correct vertebral subluxation. While it seems logical that correcting subluxations (a medical term for dislocated joints – in this case, between two vertebras) should improve one's back pain, chiropractors also claim that manipulating the spine and treating vertebral subluxation can cure various diseases and non-orthopedic maladies. In fact, the father of chiropractic care, Daniel Palmer, purportedly cured a man of chronic deafness following a spinal adjustment.[1]

Prior to my visit, Beth and I went out to dinner with a couple of our friends, and I casually mentioned I had an upcoming chiropractic visit. My friend John became very animated and related that he has regularly visited a chiropractor since high school. He said every so often, his back "goes out of whack," and he goes to see a chiropractor for a few adjustments. Before long, his back returns to normal. He gave me one warning though: "Be aware of the chiropractor when he moves in to adjust your neck." He described lying flat on an exam table with his face down. Out of the corner of his eye, he saw the doctor's feet circling around the room, and he heard the doctor's soothing voice telling him to relax. Unexpectedly, the chiropractor snuck in and performed an aggressive adjustment of John's neck. Of course, John's story only heightens my growing fears about my upcoming visit. By the morning of my visit, my back is actually feeling a bit better, and I contemplate canceling. In the end, I buck up and go.

The office is in a nondescript, single-level office complex. It is small and a bit dated compared to most doctors' offices. I fill out the requisite history form. While waiting, I notice back rests still wrapped in cellophane placed around the lobby in several chairs and in a large basket in the corner. A price of $25 is clearly labeled on each cushion. Perhaps this is a source of additional revenue – a bit chintzy if you ask me. After waiting for about 15 minutes, the receptionist calls my name, then gives me a cup and points me toward a small restroom and requests that I provide a urine sample. This must be to exclude a urinary tract infection as the cause of my back pain, because I certainly can't imagine any reason they would be performing a drug screen. I am quite sure I do not have a urinary tract infection. I contemplate confessing that I am an infectious disease doctor and based on my lack of urinary frequency, burning, or other systemic signs, I clearly don't have an infection. In the end, I decide it is best to just play along. After proudly providing the assistant with a frothy cup of warm urine, I am led to a seat in a small check-in room. To pass the time until the doctor arrives I read the flyers on the walls. I am struck by a flyer that proclaims, "We advise: NO FLU SHOTS!" The flyer lists a litany of reasons why flu shots should be avoided, citing various medical journals and specialists to support these claims. The justifications include all of the following: "It does not prevent pneumonia in older persons" (*Lancet, New England Journal of Medicine*); "5 consecutive flu shots increase the risk of developing Alzheimer's by 10X" (1997, NVIC Vaccination Conference, Hugh Fundenburg, MD); and "Studies suggest low vitamin D levels may actually be responsible for flu symptoms rather than the influenza virus!" I am flabbergasted. Two visits to alternative practitioners and two attacks on vaccination! Later, I do some research on the assertion about flu vaccination and an increased risk for Alzheimer's disease and find that the doctor who made this claim has been stripped of his medical license by the South Carolina Medical Board, and his claims have been discredited.

After about five minutes of perusing the check-in room walls, I am interrupted by the chiropractor's assistant. She takes a seat across from me and reviews my history form and confirms my complaints. She leads me into the examining/adjustment room. The assistant instructs me to get undressed and says she has some shorts for me to wear if I desire. I say, "No, I am comfortable in my underwear." After an awkward silence, she says, "Okay, why don't you just leave your pants on and strip off your shirt." Apparently, standing in my underwear is not appropriate. She steps out and I am forced to contemplate my choice of dress or undress while I wait for the doctor to come in.

As I wait for the chiropractor, I examine the walls in my new setting for additional interesting tidbits. The room is unremarkable except for a large exam table with many detachable parts and a complicated system of foot pedals for adjustment. On the wall directly opposite the door is a foam board with multiple cubbies containing roughly a hundred glass vials. Arranged in alphabetical order are various pills and powders. Most of the names are foreign to me. I recognize one labeled "thymus" and another "spleen." Apparently, these are some of the herbs and homeopathic remedies advertised in the center's brochure. On the long wall to the right of the door is a bulletin board with various postings. One is a picture showing MRI images of a person's lower spine. The images are labeled "before" and "after" decompression. The "before" shot shows a vertebral disc impinging on the spinal cord, while the "after" shot looks entirely normal. I also see an advertisement for "Estronex," a urine test that measures estrogen metabolites and claims to be able to determine a woman's risk for breast cancer. This is a bold claim and one which I sincerely doubt. I will have to research its veracity later.

After a short while, Dr. D enters the room. He instructs me to stand, step forward, and perch on one leg. He remarks that my pelvis is tilted. Apparently one side rides higher than the other. He then commands me to lie face down on the exam table and calls for the assistant. He instructs her to "loosen me up." This reminds me of a gangster telling his lackeys to soften up the victim before he comes in and extracts a confession. She spends about ten minutes attempting to relax the muscles that run along my spine. This is not an easy task. She presses with her palms, her forearms, and even her elbows. The sensation alternates between soothing and excruciating depending on where and how firmly she applies pressure. On completion, she places some warm towels on my back and calls the doctor. He has me remain lying face down. He places a few lifts under my hips and then begins to do some "adjustments." He asks me to breathe in, presses over my mid-spine, and cracks my back. Next, he sits at the foot of the table and pulls my legs. Then, he begins to circle, reminding me of a vulture sizing up its prey. I remember my friend John's comments, and I reflexively tense up despite my best efforts to remain relaxed. He moves in for the kill. He presses on my head and the side of my neck and sends a ripple of cracking up my neck. He then repeats this from the other side (not my favorite feeling). I cautiously wiggle my hands and feet. I am not paralyzed. Next, he pushes down on various portions of my spine, and when he does, the table collapses and makes a loud clunking sound. He does a few further adjustments while I lie on my side. He is done after about 15 minutes. It seems like a decent amount of hands-on care and face time with the doctor.

Dr. D then recommends an X-ray, which we will review at the next visit. He also prescribes a session on the decompression machine. He inquires whether I drink soda. When I answer in the affirmative, he gives a knowing nod of his head as if he has found the cause of all my ills. He recommends I cut out soda, but aside from this advice, he doesn't stress any other dietary restrictions. I am struck that he does not suggest any particular exercises or lifestyle changes. He doesn't even make a plug for the seat rests that are littered throughout his office.

I am next taken to a separate room for an upright X-ray of my spine. The X-ray machine appears ancient, and the staff seems somewhat blasé about the risk of radiation exposure. After the X-rays are completed, the assistant leads me to the decompression machine, which I am eager to experience after seeing the aforementioned "before" and "after" pictures. I imagine a medieval torture device, but the machine appears benign. I lie face down on a padded table, and a soft Velcro belt is placed around my waist. The belt is attached to a seemingly ancient machine that basically provides spinal traction. The theory is that it opens the spaces between the vertebrae. I spend the next ten minutes lying in a quiet room as the machine applies moderate traction to my spine. It actually feels pretty good. After a while, I am unhooked and led to the checkout counter. I arrange a follow-up visit for the following Monday.

As I exit the building, I reflect on my visit. Similar to my visit with the naturopath, I am impressed by the amount of time spent with me by both the doctor and his staff. I appreciate all the hands-on time, with the exception of having my neck cracked. I can see why people would prefer to see a chiropractor rather than an internist for their back pain. Here, it at least seems that something is being done to cure you rather than just covering up the discomfort with pain-killers. I am somewhat surprised I wasn't given instructions regarding things to avoid and perhaps some exercises to perform. With the chiropractor, as opposed to the naturopath, I seem to play little part in getting my back to improve. Also, my neck is sore. Perhaps this new pain will distract me from my lower back discomfort.

A few weeks later, I meet my friend John, and we compare notes regarding our experiences at the chiropractor. Apparently, he has been seeing an associate of Dr. D and has had a completely different experience at his visits. He says the urine I provided was not to check for a urinary tract infection, but instead to guide the practitioner's decision regarding which supplements and homeopathic remedies to prescribe. He said his practitioner, as opposed to Dr. D, spent extensive time analyzing his diet and prescribing "alternative" remedies. This sounds a bit more exciting to me, but I decide to stay with my man and give the adjustments a chance to work.

For several days after the initial visit, my neck remains sore. My lower back pain has not improved, even with the addition of daily stretching. As my second visit looms, I dread the adjustment of my neck. Does my neck really need adjusting when it's my lower back that hurts? I again contemplate canceling. At the second visit, I am taken directly to the exam room. Dr. D places the X-rays taken at the prior visit on the light box for viewing. He points out that my left pelvis is higher than my right. He suggests I might eventually require a heel lift for my shoes to even things out, but for now, he wants to see how I respond to spinal adjustments. He again instructs his assistant to "loosen me up." She keys in on the same tender spot along the mid-lower left side of my back. Fortunately, this time she is less aggressive in her torture. Dr. D returns and performs a series of adjustments similar to the first visit. I tolerate the cracking of my neck a bit better despite experiencing the same feeling of impending doom with my face down on the table as he lurks around the room. Next, I am sent to the decompression machine, which is set this time for 12 minutes with 55 pounds of tension. Once again, this is my favorite portion of the visit. I imagine my back is being transformed from the "before" image into the "after" image. Surely my imagined herniated disc is migrating back into its correct position. Dr. D checks on me when the decompression is complete. He says he would like me back in one week. I agree, but I first want to see how much of a bill I have racked up before I schedule my return.

My insurance covers chiropractic care at a second-tier level. Unlike the small co-pay I am charged when I see my primary care doctor, for the chiropractor I have to cover a $1,000 deductible before the insurance kicks in. When I finally get the bill two weeks later, I owe a total of $252.39 for the two visits. My insurance company has negotiated the price down from an original $510 total – kind of pricey, but not too bad.

As the weeks pass, I continue to suffer from stiffness in my lower back. I am underwhelmed by the results of the chiropractic treatment so far. I finally schedule a return visit a few months later, but little changes. My friends tell me not to lose faith. My brother-in-law relates his personal experience with shoulder pain, which miraculously disappeared after a single adjustment. Another friend says he achieves the most benefit from the chiropractor when he is seen for acute disabling back pain rather than for non-urgent adjustments. He relates an instance when a single adjustment helped him go from severe pain that confined him to the couch to rock climbing within a week's time. I am left to wonder.

Coincidentally, I do not have to wait long to put the acute back pain theory to the test. In a particularly vigorous day, as I attempt to reclaim my youth, I play pick-up basketball in the park followed by ice hockey at the community rink with my two eldest sons. By the evening, I can feel my back stiffening up. By the next morning, I am in crisis mode. My back pain is markedly worse, and I am walking in a stooped position. I am aging rapidly! At this rate, I will be an old man before the end of the week. I again find myself lying on the floor of my office between patients. Now is the time to go back to the chiropractor. Despite my skepticism, I am eager for some immediate relief. I give Dr. D's office a call, and I am happy to find out he can see me in just a couple of days. By the time the appointment rolls around, I need a savior.

At my visit, I tell Dr. D about my worsened condition. He gives me a nod of understanding, observes my desperate attempt to touch my toes, and then steps out while the assistant tries to relax my tightened back with massage and some warm blankets. When Dr. D returns, he is all business. He has me lie face-down on the exam table. He presses on the back of my pelvis bone and asks me to lift my left leg towards the sky while he pushes down. He does a few adjustments and then again tests my leg strength. After a few rounds of this, it appears I am able to offer more resistance. Am I actually stronger? Am I just trying harder? He explains that in response to the strain of bending over while playing hockey, my "glutes have given out." He seems quite confident the adjustments performed should make a difference. I choose this time to ask him for some exercises I might perform to assist with my recovery. I would like to play a more active role in my recovery. He blows off this question, but prescribes a visit to the physical therapist located in his office.

I am walking more upright immediately after my visit, but as the day progresses, I deteriorate to my pre-visit condition. I hold out hope for my upcoming visit to the physical therapist and a few more adjustments with Dr. D.

Only three days have passed since my most recent chiropractic adjustment. Today I have an appointment with the physical therapist. My back feels no better. I wonder whether it might be a little too early to begin physical therapy. I threw my back out only ten days ago, my lower back is as stiff as ever, and I still have to lie on my office floor between patients. I am reassured by the fact that I don't have radiating pain into my legs. I suppose this means my discs are in place, and my spinal cord is not being pinched. I decide it is better not to think like a doctor but instead, put my faith in the chiropractor. I remind myself that the purpose of this endeavor is to give alternative therapies a real shot, even when they run contrary to my own preconceived beliefs.

I meet with Sam, the physical therapist. I am prepared for a grueling workout. Although I come directly from work in my work attire, I have brought shorts and running shoes to change into. Sam tells me there is no need. I am disappointed. I came ready to work this back problem away. It appears my expectations for this visit were a bit misguided. Sam reviews my history and does a basic exam. Primarily, he observes me bend over and attempt to touch my toes, and he watches me walk. Surprisingly, he comes to the same conclusion as Dr. D. My left pelvis is higher than my right. I have never had so many people interested in the alignment of my pelvis! Rather than suggest a heel raise, he thinks the imbalance is due to tightened hip flexor muscles. He believes he can improve my hip imbalance with a few maneuvers and some exercises done in my spare time. He takes me through multiple maneuvers, not unlike those performed by the chiropractor. He pushes deeply into my left groin to the point of moderate discomfort. In the end, he seems satisfied that my pelvis is less tilted (somehow he has managed to lengthen my left leg by over an inch, or so it seems). He thinks that if I follow his prescribed exercises and stretches, I should do well. He completes the visit with a ten-minute ultrasound treatment on my lower back. The ultrasound generates a penetrating heat that helps my back muscles relax. I leave with a regimen of five different exercises I should perform several times a day. I vow to comply (hopefully, more faithfully than I did the exercises recommended by the naturopath).

Over the next four days, my family and I have a long, relaxing weekend at a condo on the shore of Lake Erie. I take it easy, avoid heavy lifting, and do the recommended exercises. I seem to be improving incrementally, but not dramatically. On my return, I have one more visit with Dr. D, the chiropractor. This last visit is the most business-like of any of the visits so far. After a short wait, Dr. D. enters the room and performs a quick exam. He spends about ten minutes with me. He does some non-aggressive adjustments. This time, he does not vigorously crack my neck. When he steps out of the room, I snoop around and I come across a poster for applied kinesiology. Included on the poster are what appear to be pressure points on the body that correspond with various body organs. Also, there is a list of therapeutic extracts, including the previously mentioned spleen, thyroid, liver, lung, etc. Here is a whole field of medicine practiced by Dr. D that he appears not to have brought into play. I wonder why. Perhaps his knowledge that I am a physician has caused him to stay in the mainstream, or maybe this is an area explored more commonly by his associates (or maybe these extracts are aerosolized and pumped into the ventilation systems of the exam rooms!).

Two weeks have passed since I wrenched my lower back, and just two days since my final visit to the chiropractor. I must admit my back pain is considerably better. I still have some slight discomfort and tightness, but it is almost back to baseline. The last time I strained my back I was an invalid for over six weeks. I am not sure what caused my rapid improvement. Was it Dr. D? Was my back strain less severe this time? Whatever the reason, it sure is nice to be walking upright again. This seems to be a good time to examine the evidence behind some of the techniques and claims asserted at my chiropractor's office.

First, let's analyze the advertisements for Estronex, which are posted throughout the chiropractor's office. This is not, strictly speaking, related to "chiropractic" care, but I do think the products a practitioner chooses to promote reflect on the type of medicine he or she practices. This test claims to help determine a woman's risk for breast cancer by measuring the levels of various "good" and "bad" estrogen metabolites in her urine. The website for this test suggests certain imbalances in these levels are associated with an increased cancer risk. The site goes even further by stating that through dietary changes, these imbalances can be corrected. Two references are cited to support these suspicious claims. After I found these articles, the first thing that struck me was that both are authored by employees of the company that produces Estronex. This is a major conflict of interest, and in my mind, confirms that any conclusion by the authors needs to be taken with a big grain of salt. The articles themselves are merely reviews rather than research articles. The larger review article espouses the urine estrogen metabolite test to "determine one's ratio [for] . . . earlier determination of cancer risk . . ." The same article, however, admits that "no conclusive data has yet to be published showing cancer incidence falls when individuals are treated with interventions that raise the ratio . . ."[2,3] The Estronex test appears to be a waste of money, and it makes me question the professionalism of the chiropractors who willingly advertise and provide such a baseless test to their female patients.

The second claim I feel compelled to investigate is the "before" and "after" MRI pictures for spinal decompression therapy. I find these claims difficult to stomach. If such a miraculously effective non-invasive procedure exists, why was this previously unknown to me? If I were the practitioner providing this simple procedure that resolves a herniated disc, I would be shouting it from the mountaintops and leading the millions of people who suffer from sciatica to the Promised Land. I suppose you detect my skepticism. One theory regarding the possible mechanism by which decompression works is that traction on the spine lowers intradiscal pressure, thereby allowing a herniated disc to return to its normal position. On the Internet, I quickly find a scathing repudiation of spinal decompression. One doctor documented (with references) ten pages of anti-decompression evidence.[4] He points to a study in the 1980s that showed intradiscal pressure actually increased with traction as the back muscles contracted to resist the traction. It appears that traction might decrease back pain, although there is no evidence it is superior to any other intervention. A review published in the journal Chiropractic and Osteopathy by Dr. Daniel in 2007 concluded, "Only limited evidence is available to warrant the routine use of non-surgical spinal decompression, particularly when many other well investigated, less expensive alternatives are available."[5] I could find no well-done studies that substantiated its use. This all jibes with my conclusion that although spinal decompression feels good and intuitively makes some sense, in the end, it has no clear benefit.

Are there any dangers associated with spinal manipulation? Is my fear of paralysis after having my neck adjusted justified? Interestingly, a systematic review of the literature published in 2007 found that spinal manipulation of the upper spine is frequently associated with mild to moderate adverse effects.[6] Additionally, spinal manipulation was associated with a small, but significant increased risk of vascular accidents, specifically vertebral artery dissection – basically tearing the lining of a major artery in the neck. I don't tend to be alarmist, but this is scary.

What about correcting vertebral subluxations? Subluxations are the misalignments of the vertebrae, which according to longstanding chiropractic theory is felt to lead to many health problems. Chiropractors seem to always be able to see subluxations on an X-ray while radiologists may find none – it makes you wonder. There is no credible scientific evidence that substantiates the association between subluxations and disease – the exception might be a large subluxation with nerve impingement and resultant back pain.[7] Therefore, Dr. Palmer's claim that he cured a man of deafness through a spinal adjustment is surely false.

Despite not agreeing with many of the claims and techniques that my chiropractor used, I admit I still found some merit in my visits. In general, Dr. D and his staff provided a lot of "hands-on" attention. Second, I liked the fact that adjustments, spinal decompression, and the prescribed physical therapy are all pro-active attempts at getting me better, unlike an internist's technique of prescribing medicines to alleviate the symptoms. I am not sure if the chiropractor made a difference, but I am feeling better, and I do feel chiropractors remain a reasonable option for the treatment of back pain provided you are aware of the potential risks. I suspect that much like traditional physicians, there are good and bad chiropractors. Mine was just okay.

## Chiropractic

**Cost of initial consultation:** $200-$350

**Cost of follow-up visits:** $75-$200

**Cost of prescribed remedies:** Varies based on practitioner. In my case, none.

**Covered by standard insurance policies:** Frequently – often second tier coverage with deductible.

**Published research:**

There are many studies evaluating spinal manipulation for a myriad of ailments. I looked at an overview of studies for the treatment of back pain and then treatment of other disorders.

A 2013 systematic review of spinal manipulative therapy (SMT) for acute lower back pain reviewed 20 randomized controlled studies and found that SMT was no more effective than sham therapy or inert interventions.[8]

Studies of SMT for chronic back pain show varied results with some in favor and some against its benefit.[9,10,11]

A 2010 review of the effectiveness of SMT concluded SMT may be beneficial for back pain, neck pain, and migraines. The authors concluded that SMT was not helpful for asthma, hypertension, and menstrual pain. It said evidence was inconclusive for fibromyalgia, sciatica, premenstrual syndrome, and temporomandibular joint disorders.[12]

# Endnotes


1 Trivieri, L. & Anderson, J.W. *Alternative medicine – the definitive guide* (2nd ed.). Ten Speed Press. 2002

2 Lord, R. & Burdette, C. Measuring urinary estrogen metabolites for cancer risk assessment. Metametrix white paper, 2006.

3 Lord, R, Bongiovannie, ND, and Bralley, JA. Estrogen metabolism and the diet-cancer connection: rationale for assessing the ratio of urinary hydroxylated estrogen metabolites. *Alternative Medicine Review,* 2002. Vol 7,(2);112-129.

4 Barrett, S. Be wary of spinal decompression therapy with VAX-D or similar devices. http://www.chirobase.org/06DD/vaxd/vaxd.html, searched on 5/2/2011.

5 Daniel, D.M. Non-surgical spinal decompression therapy: Does the scientific literature support efficacy claims made in the advertising media? *Chiropractic and Osteopathy*, 2007;15(7):1-5.

6 Ernst, E. Adverse effects of spinal manipulation: a systematic review. *J R Soc Med*, 2007:100:330-338.

7 Homola, S. Is the chiropractic subluxation theory a threat to public health? *The Scientific Review of Alternative Medicine and Aberrant Medical Practices,* Winter 2001;Vol 5. 1.

8 Rubinstein, S.M, et al. Spinal manipulative therapy for acute lower back pain: an update of the Cochrane review. *Spine*, 2013;38(3): E158-77.

9 Senna, M.K. & Machaly, S.A. Does maintained spinal manipulation therapy for chronic nonspecific low back pain result in better long-term outcome? *Spine*, 2011;36(18):1427-37.

10 Cecchi, F., et al. Spinal manipulation compared with back school and with individually delivered physiotherapy for the treatment of chronic low back pain: a randomized trial with one-year follow-up. *Clin Rehabil*, 2010;24(1):26-36.

11 Bronfort, G., et al. Supervised exercise, spinal manipulation, and home exercise for chronic low back pain: a randomized clinical trial. *Spine J*, 2011;11(7):585-98.

12 Bronfort, G. et al. Effectiveness of manual therapies: the UK evidence report. *Chiropractic & Osteopathy,* 2010;18(3): 1-33.

# Chapter 6 Flu Shots for the Boys – Mainstream Medicine

First, let me be very clear: I believe in vaccination. The benefits of vaccination far outweigh the risks. Do people occasionally develop vaccine-related side effects? Yes, but the likelihood of any major complication is vanishingly small. This is little consolation for that one-in-a-million instance where a major side effect does occur, but it is the truth. There is no relationship between autism and vaccination.[1,2,3] The assertion that vaccination causes autism has been effectively debunked. Is there still mercury in some vaccines? Yes, some flu vaccines still use very small doses of thimerasol, a mercury-containing preservative. Is there any proof or even a suggestion of an association between these vaccines and autism or other health problems? No. Despite multiple well-conducted studies demonstrating the benefits of vaccination, there is a growing undercurrent of people who refuse to be vaccinated or to have their children vaccinated. In my opinion this is foolhardy. Clearly these people have never seen a case of measles, mumps, or the complications of chickenpox. Needless to say, my wife, my kids, and I always get the recommended vaccines.

On Thursday of this week, I open a few bills, one of which just happens to be from the hospital where I work. Beth had taken our three sons for a drop-in visit with the nurse in early January to get the recommended flu shots. All three received the inhaled nasal vaccine administered by the nurse. They were in and out after just a few minutes. We thought little more about the visit. All tolerated the vaccine, and no one came down with the flu that winter. It is now eight months later. When I open the bill for this brief encounter my jaw drops. The hospital has billed our insurance company $195 for each child! This includes an $84 charge for a less than 5-minute clinic visit with the nurse, $27 for a "therapeutic service," presumably holding the nasal inhaler to each child's nose, and $84 more for "pharmacy" costs. Our insurance company has agreed to pay a somewhat lower amount, but has denied payment of the $84 "clinic visit" cost outright. Ultimately, this $84 per child has been billed to us by the hospital. That's $252 out of pocket for three flu shots. Not only am I irate, I am embarrassed to work at an establishment that could even consider this to be appropriate. We could have taken all three children to the local Walgreen's and had each immunized for $20 apiece, tops.

Needless to say, I call the toll free number for "questions about your bill." I immediately identify myself as a doctor and employee of the hospital, and ask to have my bill reviewed. The first woman I speak with is only able to parrot back to me the charges listed on the bill. She confirms that I in fact do owe $252. After I express my frustration, she connects me with her supervisor. The supervisor is sympathetic and says that she too would be shocked by such a bill. She says she will look into the matter and get back to me. Four days have passed, and I am still waiting. I am hopeful she will eventually get back to me with the matter resolved, and by "resolved," I mean that I owe no money. We will see.

The larger matter is that experiences like this add to one's disillusionment with "modern medicine." Why do my employer and I both spend hundreds of dollars a month for my health insurance if I get screwed in the end? It is no small wonder that millions of people in the U.S. and worldwide have said enough is enough and have sought alternatives for their medical care. While the costs may be fully "out of pocket" when seeing most alternative practitioners, at least you have a better idea of what you are paying for. I am not yet condoning any "alternative" modality over traditional care, but I am still early in my journey, and I can't promise what my final conclusion will be. Despite this one frustrating episode, I will continue to get my children and myself vaccinated even if it means a few inconveniences.

## Vaccination and Autism

**The controversy:** A British gastroenterologist, Dr. Andrew Wakefield, published a study of 12 patients in a leading medical journal, *The Lancet*, in 1998. The article claimed an association between children receiving the MMR (Measles-Mumps-Rubella) vaccine and a non-specific colitis that was believed to be a harbinger of autism.[4] The study has not stood the test of time. The results could not be replicated by other labs. *The Lancet* ultimately retracted the article, and ten of the twelve study authors withdrew their support for the study. A decade of subsequent research has refuted that the MMR vaccine has any connection to Autism Spectrum Disorder (ASD). Despite this, the seed had been planted, and persons continue to blame vaccines for the rise in ASD diagnoses.

The three main hypotheses that continue to be proposed for how vaccines lead to ASD are the following:

1) The combination of MMR vaccine causes autism by damaging the intestinal lining, allowing the entrance of proteins which damage the brain – Dr. Wakefield's assertion.

2) Thimerosol, an ethylmercury-containing preservative in some vaccines, is toxic to the immune system.

3) The administration of too many vaccines overwhelms the immune system.

**Published research addressing the three main hypotheseses[3]:**

1) **MMR causes autism** – The original Wakefield study was flawed by lack of control subjects, the assessments were not blinded, and the gastrointestinal symptoms did not predate autism in several of the subjects. Hence, the hypothesis that the breakdown in the intestinal lining allowing brain-damaging vaccine-related peptides to enter the brain is implausible. Subsequent studies have found no evidence of intestinal inflammation associated with MMR vaccination. Numerous ecological studies, case control studies, retrospective cohort studies, and prospective cohort studies have also found no association between MMR and autism.

2) **Thimerosol causes autism** – Thimerosol is an antibacterial compound used in multidose vaccine preparations for many years. It is not in live-virus vaccines such as MMR. Despite no data suggesting harm from thimerosol in vaccines, in 1999 the American Academy of Pediatrics recommended its removal from all vaccines given to young infants. The timing of this pronouncement, shortly after Dr. Wakefield's study in 1998, provoked concerns in parents that there was an unreported link between thimerosol in vaccines and autism. In fact, no such association exists. The concern for thimerosol causing autism is biologically implausible. The symptoms of mercury poisoning are distinct from those of autism. Multiple subsequent studies have failed to support an association between thimerosol and autism.

3) **Too many vaccines causes autism** – This idea was born from a Vaccine Injury Compensation Program regarding

a young girl with a mitochondrial enzyme deficiency whose encephalopathy worsened after multiple vaccines. It has been subsequently postulated that too many vaccines overwhelms a child's immune system, leading to an autism-inducing autoimmune response. Again, this theory is based on flawed reasoning. Vaccines do not overwhelm the immune system. Vaccinated and unvaccinated children are equally prone to infections by non-vaccine-preventable illnesses.[5] The antigenic exposure provided by vaccines is minuscule relative to the daily exposure our immune systems respond to. A more recent study confirmed that increasing exposure to antibody-stimulating proteins in vaccines in the first years of life was not related to the risk of developing ASD.[1] Additionally, autism is not an immune-mediated disease; rather, it is likely a genetic variation in our neuronal circuitry combined with environmental exposures as yet to be determined.

# Endnotes


1 Destafano, F., et al. Increasing exposure to antibody-stimulating proteins and polysaccharides in vaccines is not associated with risk of autism. *J of Pediatrics,* 2013;63(2):561-67.

2 *Immunization safety review: Vaccines and autism*. Institute of Medicine, May 14, 2004.

3 Gerber, J.S. & Offit, P.A. Vaccines and autism: a tale of shifting hypotheses. *Clin Infec Dis*, 2009;48:456-61.

4 Wakefield, A.J., et al. Ileal-lymphoid-nodular hyperplasia, non-specific colitis, and pervasive developmental disorder in children. *Lancet,* 1998; 351: 637-41.

5 Black, S.B, et al. Apparent decreased risk of invasive bacterial disease after heterologous childhood immunization. *AM J Dis Child,* 1991;145:746-9.

# Chapter 7 Me, the Porcupine – Acupuncture

Having survived my dalliances with both the naturopath and the chiropractor, I am ready to kick my alterative explorations up a notch. Acupuncture seems like the perfect next stop in my adventures. Acupuncture has been practiced in China for over 5,000 years. The basic principle of this ancient practice is the belief there is a vital life energy called "chi" present in all life forms. Chi circulates along 12 major energy pathways called meridians. These meridians are linked to specific organs and systems. There are purportedly over 1,000 acupoints along the meridians that can be stimulated to enhance the flow of chi.[1] Needles inserted into these acupoints supposedly provide pain relief and restore health. Acupuncture is used to treat a long list of conditions including both acute and chronic pain, addiction, mental disorders, and infertility. When I go online to investigate if there are any acupuncturists nearby, I am amazed to find over 40 sites in the Cleveland area. That is a lot of needles being stuck in people. Apparently, acupuncture has caught on in a big way. Before we get too far in this new endeavor, let me come clean . . . This whole concept of "chi" sounds wacky to me. I don't remember coming across these meridians when I was dissecting my cadaver in anatomy class. Despite my skepticism of "chi," my perception is that acupuncture must work for some people. I have heard testimonials of major surgeries being done using only acupuncture, rather than general anesthesia. Could this be due to the placebo effect on a massive scale, or possibly a form of hypnotism? I am not sure why it works, but it clearly has an effect for some. The question I have is, Will it do anything for me?

I schedule an appointment with a local acupuncturist, and I admit to being a bit nervous. Despite being a doctor, I am not a fan of needles, knives, or anything sharp that can cause pain. My wife can attest to this. She loves Quentin Tarantino movies, including *Kill Bill*. It is a particularly gruesome movie, which insists on following the path of every knife or sword in excruciating detail. I couldn't help but cover my eyes to shield myself from the gratuitous bloodshed. Eventually, I stopped watching, due to nausea. Adding to the fear of seeing an acupuncturist with his/her sharp needles is my aversion to anything touching my feet. My kids know this all too well and are always sneaking up on me and grabbing my feet when I am lying flat. I am terrified that the acupuncturist might actually stick a needle somewhere in my foot. From my research, this seems to be an all-too-likely possibility. According to a drawing in my reference book of the >1,000 acupoints, the feet have more than their fair share.

Despite my fears, I decide that if I am going to try acupuncture, I will do it right. Rather than see a granola-eating, hippie, Asian wannabe, I will seek out the real deal. If acupuncture comes from China, I should go to a practitioner from China. I find a Dr. Z Lin (name changed for my protection; nobody wants a mad Asian woman with needles coming after him!), who received her training at the Academy of Traditional Medicine in Beijing, China. She reportedly comes from a long lineage of traditional Chinese medical doctors and began to learn her trade as a teenager under the tutelage of her mother. Her website (yes, she has a website) has a long list of maladies that she treats, including gastrointestinal disorders, gynecologic disorders (here is one I don't have), respiratory disorders, headaches, back pain, allergies, addictions, anxiety, and shingles. This seems like the right place for me. I decide I will ask her to focus on my headaches and back pain, which amazingly are still nagging me despite my visits to a naturopath and a chiropractor. I give Dr. Z Lin a call, and I am able to make an appointment within a week.

The acupuncturist's office is located on the second floor of a nondescript office complex. I open the door of her office, and I am greeted by an empty room with two chairs against one wall and a desk against the other. There are two closed doors in the back of the room, which lead to two small exam/treatment rooms. There is little indication that I am in the right place – no visible medical texts, no flyers advertising herbal products, nothing. I sit down, and after a brief period, Dr. Lin, a short Asian woman frocked in a white doctor's coat, exits one of the two exam rooms. It appears to be a one-woman operation, no secretary, no assistant, just her. Based on the set-up and a single poster on the inside of the entrance door, I get the impression the office space is at times shared with a massotherapist who specializes in "hot rock" massage and similar therapies, but at the moment, Dr. Lin appears to be practicing alone. A second later, an elderly woman in her mid-60s exits the exam room. By eavesdropping on their conversation, I surmise she has been receiving treatment for sciatica, comes to the office on a regular basis, and is quite pleased with the results. Dr. Lin practices a fee-for-service business, which requires payment at the time of services rendered. The woman pulls out her credit card and pays on the spot. The price is $85 for an initial visit and $75 for subsequent visits.

After the woman leaves, the doctor turns her attention to me. I fill out a one-page form describing my complaints and demographic information. I briefly describe to Dr. Lin my headaches and my lower back pain. That is about it – minimal history and no physical exam. While reviewing my intake form, she notices I am a doctor, which seems to surprise her.

She then leads me into one of the treatment rooms. The room is sterile in appearance. There is an exam table in the middle of the room; an acupuncture poster on the wall showing the 12 meridians; and a counter with needles, cotton balls, alcohol swabs, and other medical equipment. I feel a bit disappointed. In picking a doctor from China who is trained in traditional Chinese practices, I expected more of an Oriental flare. I thought the doctor would be dressed in a kimono and there would be Oriental music or at least the sound of a babbling brook in the background. I expected the smell of incense to be wafting in the air and for the doctor to supplement her treatment with herbal remedies. Alas, none of this is present. Rather, Dr. Lin seems to have adopted a more "Western" approach. At least I feel rather confident that the needles will be clean!

Following Dr. Lin's instructions, I lie down on my right side with my shirt pulled up to expose my back while I face a large clock on the wall. It is one of those big round clocks with a white face and black numbers that adorn the walls of classrooms. Dr. Lin carefully places the needles into my body, about 15 in all. She first places several needles over my temples, ears, forehead and scalp. I try to stay very still, and as a result, I am not able to fully visualize the process. It feels like she inserts the needle and then flicks it to push it in further. It causes minimal discomfort, except for tightness around my scalp. She then places several needles along my mid- and lower back. These are painless. She next places a needle right in the middle of my left calf. Ouch! I feel this one. It sends a shooting, nerve-like pain along my calf. The pain quickly subsides, but I feel a bit uneasy. She next places several in the tops of my feet and ankle, but fortunately, she leaves the bottom of my feet alone. She looks up and surveys her work. "You are sweating," she says. I think to myself, "Of course I am sweating, you idiot. I am a human pin cushion. I can't move for fear of stabbing pains!" Instead I answer, "It's just my nature, I always sweat a lot." She asks if I am hot. I say that I am fine. She places a heat lamp next to my back. Now I am hot.

Dr. Lin places a small bell in front of me to ring if I need assistance. She says she will be back in 30 minutes, and that it is okay for me to fall asleep. I say "okay," and she steps out. Of course, it is more likely that pigs will fly than I will fall asleep! By nature, I am a wiggler. My friends call me the "princess and the pea" because I need perfect conditions to sleep. I generally roll from side to side every 5 minutes for 30 minutes to an hour each night before finally nodding off. No way am I sleeping now. I can feel the tightness in my scalp from the many needles and a slight discomfort emanating from my calf. Will I be able to lie still for 30 minutes? I find myself staring at the clock. "Tick, tick, tick." The minutes slowly pass as the clock provides the only sound in the room. After an eternity, Dr. Lin returns. She asks, "Do you still have a headache?" I hesitate because I actually have developed a much greater headache than when I came in. "Not sure?" she asks. I nod. "Let's stimulate you a bit," she says. She then proceeds to wiggle each needle in my scalp and in my back. I feel only a minor twinge as they are jiggled. She then steps out again. Another eternity seems to pass. Now I am not even sure when she will be coming back.

Finally, my curiosity gets the best of me. I must see what I look like. I cautiously raise my head up to try to look at my feet and legs. My movement is stopped abruptly by a sharp pain in my back. Quickly, I lie back down. My muscles are now tensed, and I am sweating profusely. I wonder if I have undone all the possible benefits. After 15 minutes, she returns. She extracts all of the needles while dabbing at the puncture sites with alcohol. She asks if my headaches usually start in my temples. I concur. She suggests that she bleed me a bit. Have I returned to the Dark Ages? Wasn't President George Washington's death hastened by bloodletting?

Of course, I say nothing. She takes a small instrument and stabs me over each of my temples and follows up with some pinching and pressure. It takes a few minutes, and I am left with only a red dot on each side of my head. It appears that I was bled less than I anticipated.

Dr. Lin is finished, and she suggests I return within one week. She says the continued treatments should provide longer and longer periods of relief. I fail to tell her that I now have a sizeable headache and my back feels unchanged. Despite this, I go ahead and arrange a visit for the following week.

Ultimately, I cancel my return visit to see Dr. Lin. As a result of my first visit, I had an intense headache that took days to resolve, and my back pain was no better. The main reason I cancel is I cannot imagine lying motionless again for 45 minutes with nothing to distract me but the ticking of a clock. Instead, I schedule a visit with a nearby acupuncturist whom I locate online. It just so happens that her office is located in the same building as my naturopath. This only deepens my suspicion that all alternative medicine practitioners are in cahoots!

Dr. Jones has clearly just relocated to this newly renovated office space. I will refer to her as Dr. Jones, although, like Dr. Lin, she really doesn't appear to hold a doctorate. The office is clean and spartan. Again, there is no receptionist, and the walls are barren of pictures. Dr. Jones appears to be a nice woman in her mid-40s. She more closely fits the hippie mold I expected from a non-Asian practitioner. She leads me into one of the two treatment rooms, and I am relieved to see a boom box in the corner and no large clocks on the wall. I am hoping music will help the session pass by more quickly. Dr. Jones spends 15 minutes taking a thorough history. She inquires about my headaches, back pain, sleep habits, and dietary habits. She asks whether I drink eight glasses of water a day. I hate this question. No one knows where the adage that one must consume at least 64 ounces of water a day comes from, but it is a myth that continues to be perpetuated by health care providers. Yes, it is important to be hydrated, but drinking beyond what your thirst requires generally just means more urine. Next thing you know, we will all be told we need eight bottles of Evian each day! She then measures the pulses in my wrists and hands by palpating three separate points on each limb. She says she is not concerned with my heart rate; instead, she is "appreciating the quality of my pulses." She is intrigued by the pulses in my left hand. She says these suggest I have "sleep difficulties." She then examines my tongue. I proudly point out I have not brushed my tongue today because I had read not to do so in one of my books. She gives me a half smile. I wonder if I have bad breath.

She has me lie face down on the table and inserts needles along my neck, mid-back, legs, and ankle region. There is no discomfort as she places the needles; in fact, I barely feel them. She puts on some relaxing music, dims the lights, and steps out. This time, I actually do come close to falling asleep. After 25 minutes she returns, removes the needles, and instructs me to lie flat on my back. This time, she inserts needles in my wrists, between my thumbs and index fingers (here I feel a short stabbing nerve pain, but it quickly dissipates), and several around my knees and ankles. She steps out again. I find it much harder to lie still this time. I have an overwhelming temptation to wiggle. After a while, I try moving my arms, and I am rewarded with a quick searing pain. "Must lie still," I tell myself. Boy, am I bored! After about five hours, which is in fact only 25 minutes, she returns. The needles come out, and I am done. At this point it dawns on me that I cannot return for more. Book be damned, I can only take two of these acupuncture sessions. Watching golf on television, playing tennis with my four-year-old, and reruns of the Lawrence Welk show all pass time faster than these visits. I, of course, do not tell this to the doctor. I will have to email or call back and cancel the scheduled follow-up.

Payment is a bit awkward. Dr. Jones informs me she only takes cash or check. I never carry checks, and only by the grace of God do I have any cash. My wife had actually put some money in my wallet that morning. Unfortunately, I only have $50 and the fee is $60. She is unfazed and pockets the money. I sheepishly offer to bring by a check for the remainder, but she states, "You are good for it. You can just pay me at your next visit." I will be mailing it in.

Once again, acupuncture has not led to a miraculous cure of my back pain. Also, the pattern of my headaches remains unchanged over the subsequent weeks. At least this time my visit did not cause a headache.

As I attempt to assess acupuncture as a discipline, let me first acknowledge I did not give acupuncture a fair shake. I only attended two sessions with two different practitioners. I have already been accosted by several of my wife's friends, who have offered testimonials regarding the benefits they experienced with acupuncture. They remind me that it is recommended that one receive multiple treatments, at least weekly at the beginning, if one wants to achieve positive results. Alas, I admit I have not done this and will not be doing this. I can handle a degree of pain; I can force feed myself handfuls of pills; I am willing to foot a large bill; I am even willing to eat vegan; but I can't handle overwhelming boredom. The needles were relatively painless (with a few exceptions), and the practitioners appeared competent, but the chore of lying completely still for up to 45 minutes at a time is beyond my capabilities. By nature, I am too fidgety and curious to lie motionless when I am chock-full of needles, doing my best imitation of a pin cushion. When my hand and wrist were impaled with needles, I was unable to overcome the desire to see how far I could move my hand without feeling searing pain. The answer – not far. When I explain this to my wife, she just rolls her eyes and treats me as if I am her fourth child.

What about those meridians? Purportedly, a team of Korean researchers in the 1960s used advanced "microdissection" techniques to look for actual anatomic structures in the body that correspond with these traditional acupuncture pathways. They claimed to have found a series of fine duct-like tubes with fluid sometimes draining in the same direction as, and at times in opposition to, known lymphatic and blood channels. More recently, researchers have used MRIs and electromyelographs in attempts to confirm that the meridians and acupoints have a biologic basis. The results of these studies are contradictory. A review of the literature performed in 2008 found several studies that showed a positive association between acupuncture points and lower electrical resistance, yet the reviewers concluded the studies were generally poor in quality.[2] A Chinese doctor, Yaun Lin, claims to have found the anatomical basis for the lines of meridians within the fascial network of the human body (basically the fibrous tissue that encases our muscles and organs).[3] I remain skeptical. As I stated earlier, the lines of chi were not apparent to me in anatomy class.

What about clinical results? Acupuncture claims to be effective for problems ranging from drug addiction to pain management during surgery. I start by Googling surgery and acupuncture. I end up viewing an incredible video of an abdominal surgery performed in China on a man using acupuncture alone in place of anesthesia. The video is a bit grainy, and the camera angles lead me to question if I might be getting scammed, but apparently he tolerated the surgery. Aside from numerous testimonials, I am unable to find any real proof that acupuncture is a viable option for surgery. Next, I look for articles supporting acupuncture for the treatment of back pain. I find a well-conducted randomized trial in a respectable journal, *The Archives of Internal Medicine,* which compared four regimens for chronic low back pain: 1) an individualized acupuncture regimen, 2) a standardized acupuncture regimen, 3) a sham regimen, and 4) a non-acupuncture based regimen where participants received the usual care that their individual physicians chose.[4] The findings: The first three groups all had similar decreases in their perceived level of dysfunction. All three of these groups, which also included the sham group, felt significantly better than the usual care group. The authors' conclusion was that tailoring needling sites and penetrating the skin appeared unimportant in eliciting therapeutic benefits. The likely conclusion is that the patients were largely experiencing a placebo phenomenon. The placebo phenomenon is response in which a placebo, or fake treatment, can improve a patient's condition because the patient has the expectation that it will be helpful.

To be fair in my analysis, I decide to include findings from the journals that focus on complementary medicine rather than just traditional medicine. This leads me to a review article published in the *Journal of Complementary Medicine* in 2004, which concludes ". . . international agreement has emerged that acupuncture appears to be effective for postoperative dental pain, postoperative nausea and vomiting, and chemotherapy-related nausea and vomiting." Beyond this, acupuncture was found to be at best "promising" for some conditions, "inconclusive or difficult to interpret" for others, and of no benefit for smoking cessation or weight loss.[5]

What are my conclusions? The jury is still out. Admittedly, my own experience was limited due to my inability to lie still. The literature supporting acupuncture is underwhelming. I know that many of you consider me the ultimate skeptic, unwilling to give any "alternative" medicine a fair day in court. I did expect the literature would have more clear evidence that acupuncture works. Despite this, I am willing to keep an open mind and possibly try acupuncture again in the future. China is a big country. Who am I to argue with the convictions of over a billion people? I don't see myself ever using acupuncture for surgical pain, but maybe, just maybe, I might try it again for my recurring headaches.

To place my acupuncture experiences in perspective, consider the following. Two weeks after my visits with the acupuncturists, I have a long delayed appointment with my dentist to have some cavities filled. I had found myself repeatedly putting off the visit for a couple of reasons. First, I am now skeptical of all healthcare practitioners, whether they practice "alternative" medicine or otherwise, and second, I haven't had a cavity in 30 years, and now I was told I have three. It just doesn't make sense. In fact, the dental hygienist was the first to look at the films and her preliminary read was that they looked fine. The dentist initially agreed, but on second glance thought she could appreciate some "shadows" representing cavities. Not real convincing. Ultimately, I succumbed to her expertise and made the follow-up appointment. I have calculated that if I ignore her advice, I might end up needing a root canal in the future, an event I would rather avoid. I hate having dental work done. Although it has been over 30 years since my last filling, I still carry a healthy dread of being drilled on. I show up for the appointment and suffer through 45 minutes of numbing, drilling, filling and general discomfort. I hate it, but in the end, I have an amazing realization . . . it is better than acupuncture!

## Acupuncture

**Cost of initial consultation:** $20-$150

**Cost of follow-up visits:** $20-$100

**Cost of prescribed remedies:** 0

**Covered by standard insurance policies:** Hit or miss. Some provide full coverage for "accepted conditions," while other insurers provide no coverage. Individual acupuncturists often leave it up to the individual to file a claim.

**Published research:**

There are many studies in the literature. Unfortunately, there are not many good studies. The best studies attempt to have a "control" by using a sham procedure to simulate the penetration of the acupuncture needle or use alternative points not related to the acupuncture map.

In 1997, NIH Consensus Conference conclusions were: Acupuncture shows evidence of efficacy for adult postoperative and chemotherapy nausea and vomiting, and for postoperative dental pain. It may be a useful adjunctive treatment for several other conditions.[6]

My personal review of the literature found possible benefit for migraines, depression, nausea, dental pain, and chronic pain.[7] No benefit for irritable bowel syndrome, hypertension, surgical anesthesia, and chronic knee pain due to arthritis.[8] There was equivocal benefit for many other conditions. Certainly the question remains: Why does acupuncture work? In the absence of proven meridians and acupoints, are we really just seeing a heightened placebo phenomenon or the response to endorphin release?

# Endnotes

1 Trivivieri, L. & Anderson, J.W. *Alternative medicine – the definitive guide* (2nd ed.). 2002.

2 Ahn, A.C., et al. Electrical properties of acupuncture points and meridians: a systematic review. Bioelectromagnetics, 2008 May;29(4):245-56.

3 Lin, Y. & Yu, B. Anatomical discovery of meridians and collaterals. Abstract presented at Fascia Congress, 2009.

4 Cherkin, D.C., et al. A randomized trial comparing acupuncture, simultated acupuncture, and the usual care for chronic lower back pain. *Arch Intern Med,* 2009. May 11;1699): 858-866.

5 Birch, S., et al. Clinical research on acupuncture. Part 1. What have reviews of the efficacy and safety of acupuncture told us so far? *J Altern Complement Med*, 2004 June:10(3):468-80.

6 NIH Consensus Conference – Acupuncture. *JAMA*, 1998;280917):1518-24.

7 Vickers, A.J., et al. Acupuncture for chronic pain – individual patient data meta-analysis. *Arch Intern Med*, 2012;172(19):1444-1453.

8 Hinman, R.S., et al. Acupuncture for chronic knee pain – a randomized clinical trial. *JAMA*, 2014:312(13):1313-1322.

# Chapter 8 Is This Hell? – Hot Yoga

One might argue whether yoga is a form of alternative medicine, but when I discuss my list of maladies in the context of the book I am writing, people invariably suggest I try yoga. I have dabbled in yoga in the past, but I have failed to truly embrace it. My wife has a series of yoga DVDs she does regularly. Over the years, I have joined her for home yoga sessions a handful of times, but that is about it. I have done enough to be familiar with terms such as "up dog" and "down dog" even when our canine, Jack, is not present. My overall impatience and my supernatural lack of flexibility have limited my excitement for yoga. Despite this, I suspect yoga might be just the thing to help with my back pain, and possibly even aid me in relaxing. With these thoughts in mind, I have decided to give yoga another go-round.

Yoga traces its origins back to ancient India. It is described as a physical, mental, and spiritual discipline in which the practitioner strives to attain a state of perfect spiritual insight and tranquility. Yoga, as practiced in the West, is largely a derivative of the Hatha system of yoga, which traces its roots back to the 15th century, but the practice did not become commonplace in the West until the early 20th century. Hatha yoga is comprised of various physical poses that have been adopted in the West of as a form of meditation and exercise.[1] Similar to other forms of alternative medicine, practitioners of yoga claim it imparts measurable benefits: improvement in post-chemotherapy nausea, decreased risk of cardiovascular disease, and improvement in general well-being, to name a few. As with all forms of alternative medicine, these claims are met with a range of responses from the general populace – from unquestioning agreement to outright skepticism. Unfortunately, a truly convincing placebo-controlled study is unlikely to ever take place. I suppose one group could be instructed in good yoga posture and the other could be instructed in bad yoga posture, but I think most skeptics would still not be convinced. The benefits of yoga are hard to quantify. How do you measure spiritual enlightenment and inner peace? In this instance, I will follow the masses. Everyone from my favorite basketball player growing up, Kareem Abdul Jabbar, to the cultural icon Madonna has done yoga. Why not me? I could use some inner peace. I also imagine an increase in balance and flexibility would be beneficial. Maybe my back pain will drift away, and I will sleep soundly through the night. We shall see.

In an attempt to limit my own embarrassment, I first do some private home yoga workouts to prepare for my public yoga debut. I start by doing my wife's yoga workouts twice a week for a month in hope of developing a minimal level of flexibility and balance. I begin with the first of three sessions on Bryan Kest's *Power Yoga* DVD. In case you are unfamiliar with Bryan Kest, he is, or at least was at the time of the filming, a thirty-something yoga master with flowing locks of brown hair, sculpted muscles, and the ability to send young women's hearts aflutter. In the video, he leads a group of young, perfectly proportioned, and impossibly flexible men and women through an increasingly challenging series of yoga sessions. He stresses the need to breathe through one's nose only, a task I find very difficult to comply with while my body quivers to hold a pose. As an added bonus, he liberally sprinkles the workouts with "pearls of wisdom" that range from sage to downright absurd.

The first obstacle I must overcome as I begin my home yoga workouts is clearing enough space in our living room to allow unimpeded movement. Our living room is a disaster zone. One might guess a tractor-trailer carrying all sorts of paraphernalia from the movie *Cars* has been upended on our living room floor. This is on account of Thayer's, my youngest son, worship of this Disney movie, combined with my wife's inability to ignore his pleas for more toys. These factors have led to the accumulation of millions of Lightning McQueen toys and their brethren. Needless to say, accidentally stepping on, or falling onto, a car does little to help me achieve the Zen state for which I strive. With some effort, I manage to carve out an area free of obstacles and lay out my wife's yoga mat.

After suffering through the banal introduction, I am finally able to get down to business. To the best of my ability, I attempt to mimic the poses performed by Bryan Kest and his limber minions. It is not an easy task. While I find the "up-dog" pose is a great stretch for my lower back, I struggle to hold the "down-dog" pose. "Down-dog" is annoying: in addition to being "one of the best shoulder stretches in all of yoga," it is supposed to be a relaxing pose to catch one's breath before moving on to the more challenging poses. For me, it is anything but relaxing. I struggle to hold even the simplest poses. I am unable to even come close to attaining some of the intended positions. I fear I am far from reaching "equanimity" as Mr. Kest recommends. Fortunately, I am home alone, and there is no one to mock me. As I struggle to mimic the limber video models, I notice a curious phenomenon. My feet are sweating profusely. In fact, I am sweating all over, but my feet seem to have sprung leaks with copious volumes of sweat pouring forth. This makes keeping my footing extremely difficult and results in my slipping and sliding across the yoga mat. Tranquility and spiritual enlightenment seem unattainable.

After a couple of weeks of practicing solitary yoga, I decide it is time to join my wife for the intermediate level

"Tone" on Kest's DVD. I have made marginal improvements. "Down-dog" is not yet a resting pose for me, but at least my tremors have diminished to mere quivering. Watching my wife perform the poses makes me realize how far I have yet to go. It appears she could be in the video herself. I take some satisfaction in surreptitiously nudging her while she is trying to hold a particularly difficult pose. When my "accidental bump" topples her over, I offer my condolences while stifling a chuckle. I say, "That's a tough one. I struggle to hold that pose too."

During this same session, we come to a particularly difficult pose. I call the pose "the turtle" because I feel like a turtle on its back. This position entails lying on your stomach and reaching back to grab your ankles – a seemingly simple maneuver that I find to be virtually impossible. Once both ankles are clasped, we are instructed to pull out with our legs and arch our back into an inverted C. I can barely move. I struggle to lift my head off the floor. Invariably I end up with my face pressed against the floor while Beth and I break into laughter at my ineptitude. Not quite the feeling of inner peace I was expecting.

After a month of home yoga has passed, my prowess still leaves much to be desired. Nevertheless, I decide it is time for my public coming out. Unfortunately, rather than attending a yoga class, I bail out. My wife has started doing a form of yoga called Bikram yoga. It appears to be catching on across the nation. I want to join her, but there is a catch. Bikram yoga, a form of "hot yoga," is performed in a room heated to around 105 degrees Fahrenheit with 40% humidity. Furthermore, the yoga class lasts 90 minutes, rather than the standard hour of most yoga classes. I am intimidated. As a result, I don't go. I let life gobble me up, and a full six months pass before I gather up the courage to confront my hot yoga demons.

In my defense, at this time in my life I decided to take a new job at the Veterans Administration hospital in Asheville, North Carolina. As a result, I felt overwhelming pressure to tie things up in Cleveland. This meant frantically completing the many medical research projects I was working on and submitting the final work for publication. Additionally, my employer filled my plate with last-minute clinical duties prior to my departure. I had little time for any extracurricular activities. Of course, my fear of "hot yoga" made abandoning my dalliance with alternative medicine all the easier.

I am now in Asheville. I came down ahead of the rest of my family in early spring. For the next few months, I will be staying in a studio apartment while I begin my job, look for a house, and wait for my wife and kids to join me. Without a wife and kids, I have infinite time to get things accomplished. I bike. I read. I cook. I even find time to confront my yoga fears. My friend Craig, whose wife is a Bikram yoga guru, calls and implores me to get "my butt in gear" and give Bikram a try. So I do.

I look online and find a Bikram yoga studio nearby. The website lists the benefits of yoga: detoxification, weight loss, building muscle, gaining flexibility, increasing energy, and improving sleep.[2] It also claims that Bikram yoga is good for healing (injuries, stress, arthritis, high blood pressure) and mental clarity. Bikram is notable for 26 poses that are done twice each session. I read through the descriptions and benefits of these standard poses. One pose, the Eagle pose, purportedly flushes one's lymph nodes and boosts the immune system. Other postures are said to balance one's metabolism and improve splenic function. In general, the claimed benefits of the practice are primarily increased flexibility, strength, and relaxation. Overall, it seems pretty reasonable.

Despite my trepidation, I sign up for a class scheduled for the next morning. I am now committed. No turning back.

I read the online recommendations for Bikram novices: Arrive early, don't eat or drink for two hours prior to class, be well-hydrated, be prepared to feel nauseated or light headed, and at all costs . . . do not leave the heated room. After reading this, I am further psyched out. I contemplate canceling. One of my new fears, in addition to passing out from dehydration or embarrassment, is that I will need to urinate. I am plagued with a nervous bladder, which leads to increased frequency of urination, particularly when I am stressed. Unfortunately, it appears to be verboten to leave the classroom unless you are in labor (not likely for me) or you can prove you are suffering from significant blood loss.

Finally the moment arrives. The yoga studio has a pleasant atmosphere. It is comprised of a narrow entry room with a few benches and a check-in desk, two changing rooms, and a large yoga studio. I sign in at the desk and take advantage of a special offer, which allows you to attend unlimited classes over the next 30 days for $60. At the very least, this commits me to coming back several times. I like to get my money's worth.

I am in luck. Two other people are attending their first class. Maybe I will not be alone in my ineptitude. The instructor gives us some basic instructions . . . don't leave the room, breathe through your nose, and just do what you can. The yoga room reminds me of a dance studio with mirrors on the walls. There are about 25-30 persons in the class. Everyone appears very fit and pleasant. The women wear skimpy, spandex outfits, as do the men. No shirts for the men. I will have 90 minutes to closely examine all my physical flaws.

The room is hot, not warm, but hot – a Florida summer day minus the breeze. I find a space for my yoga mat and towel and then escape back outside the studio. I plan on limiting my heat exposure as much as possible. I want to maximize my chances of survival. I monitor the clock, and when there are only two minutes left, I run to the bathroom one last time and then dash back into class just as it is ready to begin.

Over the ensuing 90 minutes, the instructor leads us through the standard 26 poses, most of them done twice. Many of the poses are not too outlandishly difficult, although I am unable to do a lot of them. My poses however, bear little resemblance to the postures assumed by the veteran yoga masters. I quickly note three things: I am the least flexible person; I have the worst balance; and I sweat more than anyone else. I am surely a distraction to my fellow yogis. I repeatedly topple from my attempted poses, even poses whose main challenge is to remain balanced while standing on one leg. Also, I am sweating like a banshee! I am embarrassed by the rivulets of sweat flowing off of me. The steady patter of my sweat on the yoga mat is magnified in my ears. Midway through the class, I wonder if I will make it. I am losing water rapidly, much quicker than I can replace it through my furtive sips of water from my water bottle. Despite my determination to do otherwise, I am forced to take a few breaks during the class. These breaks entail lying on my back and staring at the ceiling. They are only mildly refreshing in the virtual sauna.

I am amused by the pearls of wisdom doled out by our instructor, which I later learn are all part of the Bikram dogma. One particular statement vexes me. We are instructed to "breathe through your nose rather than your mouth as this gets more oxygen to your lungs." I don't remember being taught this in medical school. Later, I research this claim. I Google "mouth breathing versus nose breathing" and get over 100 hits. The vast majority of these quasi-scientific links tout the health benefits of nose breathing. Benefits range from improved warming and filtration of the air to social acceptance. I even find a possible mechanism whereby nose breathing might actually help your lungs extract more oxygen: "Because the nostrils are smaller than the mouth, air exhaled through the nose creates back pressure when one exhales. It slows the air escape so the lungs have more time to extract oxygen from them. When there is proper oxygen-carbon dioxide exchange, the blood will maintain a balanced pH. If carbon dioxide is lost too quickly, as in mouth breathing, oxygen absorption is decreased."[3] A plausible explanation although I doubt it is well rooted in science.

When stretching to the side, we are instructed to feel the stretch from "the outside to the inside from the skin, to the muscles, to the bones." At one point, while flexing our necks, we are told this "stimulates our thyroid, parathyroid, and pineal glands." The last time I checked, my pineal gland was encased in my skull and not very easy to compress. Certain poses and stretches are deemed to be good for digestion. One stretch even massages the ascending colon. Most of these quotes are more amusing than factual.

Somehow, I survive to the end. As the class winds down, my muscles are starting to cramp, and I am light-headed. I happily drag myself and my sweat-saturated towels from the class. I am wiped out the rest of the day, but I have a feeling of accomplishment and despite my skeptical opinion of our instructor's quips, yoga makes me feel good. Perhaps I am feeling the equivalent of a "runner's high." I am encouraged that yoga will improve my flexibility and my back and help me slow down. I look forward to the next class . . . as long as it is not tomorrow.

My next session two days later goes well. I am less anxious and better prepared. I have a different instructor, but the class is almost a carbon copy of the first . . . with much of the same dialogue. We massage our colons, stimulate our thyroids, and stretch until we can feel it in our "skin, muscles, tendons, bones." I go to bed feeling great.

My third class is brutal. I have an annoying male instructor, who takes an unwanted interest in me. He repeatedly tells me to deepen my stretches and to hold my poses longer. I feel nauseated in the heat. The room is crowded, and as a result, I am unable to position myself for an unobstructed view in the mirror. I am even less flexible than usual (imagine a board), and I have no balance. No Zen state for me today.

I am at my fourth class, and less than a week has passed since I started my Bikram experience. I am impressed with my commitment. Class starts at eight in the morning. I am concerned whether I will be adequately hydrated for class (the instructors and participants obsess about what and how much water they drink). I did a twenty-mile bike ride last night. As a precaution, I drank several large glasses of water in the evening. As a result, I was up every two hours going to the bathroom. It reminds me of the time Beth and I climbed Mt. Kilimanjaro in Tanzania. After the first day of hiking, a fellow climber offered us some Diamox she had been prescribed to prevent altitude sickness. Diamox is a diuretic, which in theory will alkalinize your blood and make you more tolerant of high altitudes. The catch, of course, is that it is a diuretic, which makes you urinate. Unfortunately, being well-hydrated and well-rested are also important, and probably more so, in preventing altitude sickness. I took the diuretic just before bedtime, and as a result, I was up all night. I found myself repeatedly being awakened by my full bladder. Then, I would carefully step over my fellow climbers, who were all happily asleep, to go outside our A-frame hut to pee. By the morning, I was wiped out. Common sense is apparently not one of my strong points. Needless to say, I suffered from altitude sickness on Kilimanjaro's peak, but I did make it to the top.

Back to yoga. As I said, I am poorly rested, but hydrated. I have staked out my favorite spot, close to the front mirror, so that no one can block my view and distract my concentration. My favorite pose is “Savasana,” otherwise known as the Dead Body Pose or Corpse Pose. Basically, it involves lying flat on one’s back with your feet together. In some respects, I even struggle with this pose. During Savasana, one is instructed to lie perfectly still and shut out all external thoughts. Neither of these tasks is among my strengths. I am always twitching and wiping the pooled sweat from my eyes. I try to focus on a water stain on the ceiling, but it is not easy. Today, my back is stiff from the prior classes, and I am forced to resort to modified sit-ups recommended for those with bad backs. Somehow, I manage to survive again.

I return a mere three days later, this time a 6:30 p.m. class right after work. The class goes smoothly. Again, I am the least limber person in the class. One comical thing occurs . . . the person next to me is a man of about my age. Midway through the class, he grabs a tissue from a tissue box on the floor in front of us and blows his nose. A few minutes later, I have the urge to blow my nose (likely because of the sweat clogging it from some downward position). I grab what appears to be the last tissue in the box and blow my nose. The tissue seems a bit strange – sort of crumpled and soggy. I realize I have reused the same tissue the man next to me had placed back in the now empty box. He does not initially comprehend what I have done, but he and I both realize simultaneously what has occurred . . . disgusting. We exchange looks of mortification, but then stoically and silently continue onward.

I find one problem with the late class. We don’t finish until 8 p.m., and I don’t get home until a half hour later. After sweating so profusely, I am severely dehydrated. Once I get home, I do not have much time to rehydrate prior to going to bed. Even if I had the time, I don’t want to drink too much and be up all night. The result . . . I am plagued by severe muscle cramps in my feet and calves throughout the night. They are so painful I am afraid to relax and go to sleep. I get up repeatedly to hydrate, eat a banana, and then potato chips. In the end, I get very little sleep and wake up with a headache. At least this once, yoga does not seem to be helping in my quest for nirvana. It has worsened my back pain, given me a headache, and led to a night of insomnia. Not to worry, I am in this for the long haul. Namaste.

Much like the chiropractor and the naturopath I visited, the yoga studio endorses various products. I am intrigued by its promotion of Kangen water, an alkaline-ionized water. The yoga studio appears to be in cahoots with the water distributor. Posted throughout the yoga studio are flyers for this Kangen water, which is available at a shop next door. The flyers claim this water has the seal of approval of the Japanese equivalent of the FDA. They show a picture of a person's blood smear with clumped red blood cells. A second picture illustrates the same person's red blood cells unclumped after the person regularly drank the alkaline water. Later, when I log onto the local Bikram website for more information about Kangen water, I learn another feature of this special water is that it is "microclustered." The site claims that "after passing through an electric current of 230 watts, the number of water molecules has been reduced from a cluster of 12-15 molecules to 5. It is literally "wetter" water and can be absorbed into our tissues 5 times more efficiently."[4] Wetter water, are you kidding me?!

This all sounds like total hooey. Once this "alkaline" water hits my acidic stomach, it could possibly act like an antacid, but more likely, it is no different than everyday tap water. Even Dr. Andrew Weil, a medical doctor, naturopath and proponent of holistic health, says the health claims for ionized and alkaline waters are "bogus."[5] Nevertheless, the yoga minions flock to the water cooler to refill, and many pay extra for monthly delivery of this special water.

Over the next two weeks, I continue to go to Bikram yoga about every third day. I become attuned to the ritual: 26 poses done in the same order, breathing through my nose, quick relaxation and slowing of the heart rate during the Savasana pose. I am now familiar with most of the poses. I move in unison with my fellow yoga disciples. At times, I feel I have joined a cult. Despite this, I cannot complain about the way it makes me feel. My back and joints feel better, and I find the ritualized routine relaxing. Don't be fooled into thinking I buy into all the hoopla. I still don't believe I have "memories in my spine" that need to be released, I do not get the "equivalent of eight hours relaxation" from a single pose, and I doubt that flexing my neck during certain postures has any impact on my pineal gland. Aside from these doubts, I do think yoga, and Bikram yoga in particular, provides many positive benefits for both one's body and spirit.

Struck by the cultish feel of Bikram yoga and the regimented classes, I am compelled to do a little research on its founder. Bikram Choudhury devised and copyrighted a series of yoga poses, which stem from his experiences practicing Hatha yoga as a youth in India. He won several yoga championships as a child. At age 20, his yoga career was almost derailed when he suffered a severe knee injury while lifting weights. The story goes that the doctors wondered whether he would be able to walk again, but Bikram took matters into his own hands, and through yoga, completely recovered six months later.[6] In the early 1970s, he opened his first yoga studios in the United States. His success has not been without some controversy. He has made several unfounded claims such as: participation in NASA research, instruction of past US presidents, and mentorship of the Beatles. Despite these background controversies, his regimen of yoga is widely popular. There are thousands of Bikram-trained yoga instructors, who pay upwards of $11,000 for their Bikram certification, leading millions through the same 26 poses in Bikram yoga studios across the world.[7] It appears Bikram teachers, as part of their training, are compelled to learn and then promote some amazing benefits of each yoga pose that are generally unfounded. Sure, the Eagle Pose, in which you wind your arms and legs into a difficult contortion while squatting down, strengthens your muscles and works on balance, but does it really improve lymphatic flow or boost your immune system? I think not, and I can find no evidence-based literature that says otherwise.

I have finished one month of regular attendance at Bikram yoga, twelve sessions in all. I give it double thumbs up. My body feels better than it has in a long time. I am sleeping well. The biggest drawback for me is the time required. A 90-minute class requires over two hours of my day. This is something I have been able to accomplish while my family is still in Cleveland and I am alone in Asheville, but it will be hard to sustain when we are all together. I hope to continue to attend classes, but on a more limited basis . . . maybe once a week.

## Yoga

**Cost of class:** $16 (Bikram in Asheville, NC), $0-$20 (from home exercise to studio)

**Covered by standard insurance policies:** No

**Published research:** I focused my evaluation on three main areas: treatment of lower back pain, joint pain, and other conditions. There are a lot of studies that have been done, but the majority of these were not quality studies. One limitation is that a true placebo or sham comparison group is lacking.

Chronic lower back pain:

-Randomized controlled studies: Yoga as a therapy for chronic lower back pain led to improved functional disability and less pain, although it was not better than conventional stretching exercises.[8,9,10]

-Review studies: There is modest evidence supporting yoga as an effective strategy for chronic lower back pain. The balance of studies shows yoga to be superior to usual care, education, and conventional therapeutic exercises. The findings suggest benefit, but are not conclusive.[11,12]

Neck pain, osteoarthritis, and other joint diseases:

-Randomized controlled studies: Yoga effectively reduced chronic neck pain and associated disability. Yoga was better than therapeutic exercise for osteoarthritis of the knees.[13,14]

-Review study: There was minimal evidence supporting yoga for the management of rheumatic diseases such as fibromyalgia, osteoarthritis, and rheumatoid arthritis.[15]

Other conditions:

-Yoga has shown possible, but not convincing, benefit for the following conditions: balance in the elderly, stroke patients, polycystic ovarian syndrome, post-traumatic stress disorder, smoking cessation, menopausal symptoms, schizophrenia, eating disorders, and asthma. There is no support for yoga for the prevention of coronary heart disease.

# Endnotes


1 http://www.americanyogaassociation.org/general.html
2 http://hotyogaasheville.com/index.php/about-us/postures-a-benefits
3 http://www.breathing.com/articles/nose-breathing.htm
4 http://hotyogaasheville.com/index.php/kangen-water
5 http://www.drweil.com/drw/u/QAA400790/Is-Kangen-Water-Healthful.html
6 Susman, J. *Your karma ran over my dogma: Bikram yoga and the (im)possibilities of copyrighting yoga.* 25 Loy. L.A. Ent. L. Rev, 245 (2004).
7 http://www.bikramyoga.com/TeacherTraining/Admissionfees.php
8 Tilbrook, N.E., et al. Yoga for chronic low back pain: a randomized trial. *Ann Intern Med,* 2011;155(9):569-78.
9 Sherman, K.J., et al. A randomized trial comparing yoga, stretching, and a self-care book for chronic low back pain. *Arch Intern Med,* 2011;171(22):2019-26.
10 Williams, K., et al. Evaluation of the effectiveness and efficacy of Iyengar yoga therapy on chronic low back pain. *Spine,* 2009;34(19):2066-76.
11 Cramer, H., et al. A systematic review and meta-analysis of yoga for low back pain. *Clin J Pain,* 2013;29(5):450-60.
12 Posadzki, P. & Ernst, E. Yoga for low back pain: a systematic review of randomized clinical trials. *Clin Rheumatol*, 2011;30(9):1257-62.
13 Cramer, H., et al. Randomized-controlled trial comparing yoga and home-based exercise for chronic neck pain. *Clin J Pain,* 2013;29(3): 216-23.
14 Ebnezar, J., et al. Effects of an integrated approach of hatha yoga therapy on functional disability, pain, and flexibility in osteoarthritis of the knee joint: a randomized controlled study. *J Altern Complement Med,* 2012;18(5):463-72.
15 Cramer, H., et al. Yoga for rheumatic diseases: a systematic review. *Rheumatology,* (Oxford) 2013;52(11):2025-30.

# Chapter 9 At One with the Earth – Barefoot Running

I am not a runner . . . at least not at this moment. Despite once showing great promise, I have long given up being a regular runner. In my youth a bright running future lay ahead of me. As a ten-year-old, I dominated the track and field events at summer camp; I was on the high school track team as a freshman; and I logged a few half marathons in my late 20s and 30s. Alas, as I age, the wheels are starting to fall off. Now anytime I run, I instantly feel pain in my lower back, knees, and feet. My joints lack sufficient cartilage to soften the blows. Plantar fasciitis, the dreaded runner's malady, plagues me. I figure my deteriorating condition is just the norm for an aging, 6 foot 3 inch body. People like me are not meant to be runners – basketball players maybe, but not runners. Too bad, because I have always felt running is the easiest way to get a quick fix of exercise. I love that, unlike other sports that require expensive equipment or preparation, I can lace up my shoes and be ready to go. Back in my running days, when I traveled to a new city for a conference, I would drop off my bags on arrival and go for a run to catch my bearings, open up my lungs, and clean out the pipes. Heck, I was competing in triathlons only ten years ago and having no problems.

All that changed a few years back when I began to have problems in my large joints. Now my lower back constantly aches. The aches progress to a true disability once or twice a year. My knees lack cushion. I can hear them grinding when I ride my bike or perform a maneuver as simple as kneeling down. My heels and bunions scream out in protest after any prolonged pounding that comes with an activity such as basketball or running. As a result, I am confined to biking, elliptical machines, yoga, and a few other endeavors that involve minimal impact. I have not fully ruled out competing in a triathlon again, but if I do, I will focus my training on the swimming and the cycling. I will run as little as possible until the day of the race and then I will just plan on suffering during the third leg of the triathlon. Despite my holding this grim outlook for my running future, new information has started to change my perspective. Maybe there is still hope for the running man deep within me.

I am intrigued by all things African. I read a review of a book called *Running with the Kenyans* and ask my wife to pick it up for me at the library. Instead, she accidentally picks up the audio book *Born to Run* by Christopher McDougall. I am too lazy to exchange it, and with some long drives ahead shuttling my middle son to Greenville, South Carolina, for his hockey games, I start listening to *Born to Run.* What a story! The author intertwines his own personal quest to recapture the joy of running with the story of an indigenous Mexican tribe, the Tarahumara, who have formed a society with running at its core. Along the way, he makes a strong case that, from an evolutionary perspective, man is built for running. The soles of our feet are covered with nerve endings to respond to the earth's surface, we sweat to regulate our temperature during exertion, and we have Achilles tendons to assist with strong strides. In short, we are "born to run." He also makes a convincing argument that high-priced running shoes have changed our natural running form from a mid-foot strike to an unnatural heel strike. The corollary is that this change has led to a lot of the maladies that plague many regular runners, including myself. The author leads the reader to the conclusion we should all be running barefoot, or at least be heading in this direction. He has convinced me to shed my orthotic inserts and give minimalism a try. What do I have to lose? I certainly won't be running any marathons if I continue with my current practices. I discuss my plan with my friends. Their reactions range from encouragement (meaning they also read *Born to Run*), to rolling their eyes, to downright ridicule (my doctor friends). All are in agreement: If I am going to embark on this experiment, I need to start slowly. My feet have had the past 45 years to atrophy, and I am sure my use of orthotic shoe inserts for the past eight years has further exacerbated this weakness.

I devise the following plan: I will chuck the inserts and start walking barefoot around the house and in the grassy portions of our yard for the next few weeks. I will then purchase some minimalist running shoes such as the Vibram Fivefingers. Next, I will incorporate short runs into my exercise regimen, which currently consists of biking to work and twice weekly gym workouts. As I gain foot strength, I will slowly ramp up the running. What is the worst that can happen? According to my doctor friends . . . a lot: stress fractures, Achilles strain, and calf injuries. We will see. If all goes well, I will even consider some type of short race, preferably not on pavement. I don't foresee any marathons in my future, but who knows?

For the past three weeks, I have walked barefoot around the house. For some, this may not seem like much, but for those of us with plantar fasciitis, it is a big accomplishment. It is going well. Being barefoot makes me feel closer with the earth. Surprisingly, my heels are not hurting like they have in the past. I research buying a pair of minimalist shoes. The Vibram Fivefingers appears to be closest to being barefoot, while still providing a modicum of protection. Unfortunately, the cost is $100 and up, and determining the right size online is a bit tricky. Rather than buying online, or at a "big box" store, I decide to "go local," a catchy phrase that permeates

Asheville to drum up support for local businesses. I choose a cool-looking dedicated running store near my house. It is a short visit. The saleswoman is ready to assist me before I have fully entered the front door. Now this is customer service. I ask if they carry any of the Vibram Fivefingers shoes, and she gives me a look that suggests I am crazy, and then after composing herself, kindly says they no longer carry the brand. She says the Vibrams were the hot shoes about five years ago, but then interest petered out. Instead, the store is stocked wall to wall with the latest in foot stabilization and motion control technology. There are a few "minimalist" shoes, but no Vibrams. She gives me a great tip. She recalls seeing some for sale at a nearby second-hand sports store. I rush downtown. I am a sucker for second-hand gear stores, and I love any excuse to browse around. The last time I did so, I drove home with a "new" canoe on the top of my car, much to my wife's chagrin. She had mentioned something about a budget we were supposed to be following. Budget, smudget. Who can pass up a "gently used" whitewater canoe for only $600? Well, this time is different because I now have a purpose. I will find pair of Vibram Fivefingers come hell or high water. I am not disappointed. In the shoe section, I find about ten pairs of the foot-shaped shoes, and one is my size. Fortunately, they have a special Vibram foot measuring device on the floor. I ask the salesperson if they have any more in my size. His eyes light up. There is a whole box in the back. He comes out with a box filled with Vibram shoes. I am impressed the store has over fifty pairs in stock. He corrects me and says, "Oh no, we have many more. These are just the ones in your size." Apparently, Vibram has offloaded their excess supply at clearance prices to the second-hand store. I suppose this might trigger a warning signal to some, but instead I am in rapture. A whole box of half-price Vibrams just for me! I pick out the pair that looks best for running on trails. I then sit down and try to put them on. Not easy. It appears these foot-shaped shoes are made for people with perfect, straight, conventional feet, not my craggy, cracked, deformed monstrosities. I have huge bunions, and none of my toes are straight. Nevertheless, I attempt to get the shoes on my feet, but after about ten minutes of pushing and pulling and re-directing, I give up. I decide this is a task better to be done at home, away from prying eyes. I purchase a pair for $49, signaling the true beginning of my new experiment.

My plan is to walk around in the shoes at first and acclimate my feet to their new friends. Sitting on the edge of my bed, I begin the task of putting these "foot gloves" on my feet. The angles of my feet are clearly at odds with the nice straight toe slots of the shoes. After about fifteen minutes of grunting and a few choice curse words, I succeed in getting the Vibrams onto my feet. They feel strange, yet curiously invigorating. I spend the rest of the afternoon traipsing around our house and yard "virtually" barefoot. I even shoot basketball with my son on our asphalt driveway (keeping my jump shots to a minimum). In the yard or the house, they feel great. I am not sure I can say the same about on asphalt. I decide my first runs will definitely have to be on a more forgiving surface.

The next day, I drive to the top of our mountain to a trail that parallels the Blue Ridge Parkway. It is a single track dirt trail with rocks and roots – an ideal surface for me to try out my new shoes. My plan is to start very slowly, maybe only a mile or two, to make sure I don't get injured right off the bat. As a precaution against going too fast, I bring our dog, Jack, whom we rescued from the pound many years ago. She is part Border Collie and part something small, possibly Chihuahua. Jack was once quite spry, but those days are past. She has lost an eye to glaucoma, and her remaining eye is suspect.

Additionally, her hearing is poor. Despite her maladies and her old age, pushing 14, she is fiercely loyal and loves to go for a romp in the woods. Nowadays, I keep her on a leash to prevent her from wandering off the trail and getting lost, or possibly falling off a cliff.

It has been raining off and on all day, so we have the trail mostly to ourselves. Jack and I start off at a slow pace. After the first quarter mile, Jack trails behind me on the leash, and I admonish her to keep up. I carefully pick my way along the trail, which is covered with roots and quite a few rocks. I imagine this must be similar to the paths the Tarahumara run on. I feel nimble in my new shoes as I hop from rock to rock with gratifying stretches of soft dirt in between. Despite the protection of the Vibrams, stepping on a sharp rock still feels like stepping on a sharp rock. Not much shock absorption going on. We run for about a mile and then walk back to the car on the parkway. Not too bad for a first go around.

Later that week, I run one mile on the treadmill at the local YMCA. I feel fleet of foot in the Vibrams. I also kind of like the stares I get from my fellow Ashevillians. Anything different in Asheville is cool. So I strut around the Y with my Vibrams on feeling like a trendsetter. In reality, this trend has already passed, but I am none the wiser. I am a bit wary of dropping a weight on my foot while in the weight lifting section of the gym, but I survive without a mishap.

I manage to squeeze in a couple more one-milers on the treadmill the following week. I notice some soreness in my calves near the end of my runs, but other than this, I am happy with my progress. My back is not bothering me, and my plantar fasciitis remains at bay. I am doing my best to warm up before my runs and to stretch gently afterwards. I decide it is time to go a bit farther. I run a couple of miles on a greenway next to the French Broad River, where I have the sensation of being a kid again, running barefoot in the grass.

This is wonderful. Sign me up for the New York City marathon. All is well except for a bit of nagging tenderness in my calf, which is apparent only at the end of my run.

One week later, I am in New York City, not for a marathon, but for an infectious diseases conference. I am excited to go out for a run and scout my surroundings. Like the good old days, I am able to get a quick fix of exercise and learn the lay of the land. I pull on my Vibrams and head off in the direction of Central Park. Unlike my prior runs, I am running on concrete. By the time I cover the distance of one mile and reach Central Park, I am forced to stop. I feel a sharp pain in my right calf that I am unable to shake. I hobble back to my hotel room. Over the next few days, I also notice my left knee hurts. This knee has bothered me in the past, but it has never been truly limiting. My right calf remains sore. I must have pulled a muscle. I feel like an old man. I try not to blame the Vibrams, but the thought that they may be culpable is creeping into my mind. Concrete and barefoot running are not a good combination.

After returning from NYC, I decide to take a few weeks off from running to see if I can heal my injuries. I focus on riding my bike and stretching. After three weeks of this, my calf pain has fully resolved, but my left knee still plagues me. I have pain along the inner aspect of my knee and a bit of swelling. If I flex my knee any significant amount, I feel sharp pain. I continue to stretch. I ice my knee in the evenings and take regular ibuprofen. After three more weeks pass, I am no better, maybe worse. My goal of running a 5K race this summer, or ever, appears to be a pipe dream. I am beginning to contemplate the need to see an orthopedic doctor. I hate going to see doctors . . . the inconvenience, the waiting, the cost. Of all traditional doctors, orthopedic doctors possibly scare me the most. As an infectious diseases doctor, one of my responsibilities is caring for all the persons who have developed infections after orthopedic surgery. Unfortunately, these complications are not uncommon.

Rather than doing the sensible thing, I take matters into my own hands. I perform a common act that instills fear in doctors everywhere: I research my condition on the Internet. My research combined with a brief discussion with a physician's assistant, who had previously worked with an orthopedic doctor, leads to a self-diagnosis of tendonitis of my semimembranosis or semitendinosis tendon. I find a treatment plan on the Internet for this condition, and I am ready to self-heal. Basically, I shut it down with more rest, ice, and ibuprofen. After a week, I progress to gradual strengthening exercises. I am slowly improving. After a few more weeks, I am able to resume my normal activities, and I am relatively pain free. Interestingly, I find myself choosing to wear my old thick-soled running shoes. I want nothing to do with my Vibrams. I am not willing to risk my recent recovery, and with it, a regained ability to play with my kids. My experiment with barefoot running has come to an end.

Despite my failed trial of barefoot running, I continue to believe in the principles expounded in *Born to Run*. However, the jury still seems to be out regarding the benefits of minimalist running. Daniel Lieberman, a Harvard researcher, gave credence to supporters of barefoot running with an article published in *Nature* magazine (a prestigious peer-reviewed publication) in 2010. Lieberman, through a series of elegant experiments and undecipherable equations, came to the conclusion that barefoot endurance runners preferentially land on their fore-foot or mid-foot when running, while most persons wearing running shoes tend to land on their heel (rear-foot). He found that barefoot runners with fore-foot striking generate smaller collision forces with the ground than those wearing shoes, who tend to employ a rear-foot strike. He surmised that fore-foot running is more natural and may protect against impact-related injuries, which are common among runners. These findings seem to be supported by an online survey that found barefoot and minimalist shoe wearers reporting 3.41 times fewer injuries than their traditionally shod brethren.[1] The fire in favor of barefoot running was further stoked by a publication that showed running with shoes versus running barefoot required a greater rate of oxygen consumption.[2] Hence, barefoot running uses less energy. If it sounds like the debate has been resolved, think again.

A more recent study by researchers at University of Massachusetts Amherst directly contradicts Hanson's findings. It found heel-striking to be a more physiologically economical running form, by far.[3] Additionally, a survey of runners who had tried barefoot-style shoes found 32% had suffered injuries that they attributed to the new footwear.[4]

Alas, what is one to believe? Regardless of the naysayers, I believe barefoot running can work. It did not work for me because I rediscovered it too late in my life. My feet have had the past 45 years to atrophy. As a result of fancy shoes with "balance stabilization" and "motion control," my foot muscles have lost the will to do these tasks on their own. It is too late to recapture my youth. In my next life, I will eschew padded shoes and embrace minimalism from the onset.

Of note, since I began my experiment with minimalist running, the running community, or at least the sellers of running shoes, seem to have come full circle and are now promoting new shoes with extra cushion, such as Hokas. Minimalist shoes still have a place on the shelves, but so do these moon boots. I am not sure if science is driving the changes. It seems more likely marketing is driving the science.

## Barefoot/ Minimalist Running

**Cost:** Depends on the shoes, or lack thereof. Range $0-$200

**Published research**

I focused on two issues:

1) Is barefoot/minimalist running associated with improved performance?

Improved performance: Articles by Lieberman and Hanson suggest "yes." Article by Gruber says "no."

2) Does barefoot/minimalist running lead to more or fewer injuries than running in traditional running shoes?

Fewer injuries: Article by Goss says "yes." Article by Reynolds suggests "no."

# Endnotes


1 Goss, D.L. & Gross, M.T. Relationships among self-reported shoe type, foot strike pattern, and injury incidence. *US Army Med Dep J,* 2012:25-30.

2 Hanson, N.J., et al. Oxygen cost of running barefoot vs. running shod. *Int J Sports Med,* 2011;32:401-406.

3 Gruber, A.H., et al. Economy and rate of carbohydrate oxidation during running with rearfoot and forefoot strike patterns. *J Appl Physiol,* 2013;115(2):194-201.

4 Reynolds, G. Is barefoot-style running best? New studies cast doubt. Well.blogs.nytimes.com. *Phys Ed,* June 5, 2013.

# Chapter 10 I Kneed Some Help – Orthopedics

Months have passed since my failed experiment with barefoot running, and my left knee is still bothering me. Despite giving up running altogether, my knee is showing no signs of improvement. I have tried resting it, icing it, stretching it, and strengthening it, all to no avail. Sadly, my knee pain has put a definite crimp in my activities. On the bright side, my kids see some advantage to their father being crippled. Though my oldest son, Connor, takes pleasure in our frequent family hikes, the younger two boys, David and Thayer, want nothing to do with "aimless" walks in the woods. My older sister has dubbed these types of family activities as "Forced Family fun" or "FFF" for short. When we were children, our parents took us on frequent outdoor family outings. Therefore, both my sister and I now feel it is our duty to inflict the same on our own children. While the younger boys are gleeful that my injured knee has curtailed our family hikes, they do not like that I am unable to play basketball, soccer, or tennis with them. Additionally, Thayer, our "baby," resents not getting his regular piggyback rides. I understand their complaints. I too want to be able to perform my full daddy duties. I decide my knee problem is too serious to be addressed by an alternative practitioner. So, I instead revisit mainstream medicine. I will go to an orthopedic surgeon.

This is not a hastily made decision. I have put off seeing an orthopedist for several months. A colleague of mine finally convinces me to take action. Mike, a gastroenterologist and avid cyclist, says he had the same problem with his knee and was diagnosed with a tear of his meniscal ligament. He too had been reluctant to have surgery, but when he finally went through with it, he was very satisfied with the results. Within a month he was back to his regular activities, pain free. He gave me the name of his orthopedist, and I booked an appointment.

Dr. J has an office close to the Mission Hospital in downtown Asheville. After a short wait in a typical waiting room, I am escorted to an exam room. The nurse offers me a gown to change into. I decline. Knowing that I am a physician, she does not press the issue. I have on loose fitting pants that easily roll up past my knee, so I figure why bother. Additionally, I always hate meeting the doctor while stripped down to my underwear or in a silly-looking gown. It makes you feel inferior. I try to take this into account with my own patients. I never ask the patient to be undressed prior to my first sitting down with them to exchange greetings and to listen to their concerns. Hopefully, this allows them to maintain some of their dignity, despite the subsequent medical exam.

After about ten minutes of waiting in the exam room, Dr. J knocks on the door and then enters. He is cordial and exchanges a few pleasantries before getting down to business. He takes a brief history and then has me pull up my pants so he can examine my knee. He does a few quick maneuvers to check for joint instability or focal points of pain. He notes that I have a small knee effusion (fluid on my knee). Although he is unable to elicit any other clear findings, he is suspicious I may have a meniscal tear. He suggests we arrange for an MRI of my knee. He gives me the option of following up to discuss the results, or just talking on the phone after the MRI has been completed. I chose the second option. He gets up to leave. I had only about ten minutes of face time with the doctor, but I am satisfied. I smugly remind myself that I had come to the same diagnosis.

One week later, I have the MRI. The radiologist interprets it on the spot and confirms that my left medial meniscal ligament is torn. He shows me the pictures. My ligament looks like a frayed rope, much different from the flat and smooth ligaments in the knee model in Dr. J's office. Later that afternoon, I contact Dr. J via phone, and he recommends that I be scheduled for arthroscopic partial meniscectomy. I agree, and a few calls later I am set up for surgery.

I don't question the decision to proceed with surgery. I have already done my own self-prescribed physical therapy without results. I am eager to finally have a definitive fix of my knee so I can resume normal activities. Sadly, running will not be one of those activities. Sorry, Vibram Fivefingers, I will not be taking you out for any more jogs. Why should I question surgery, which is mainstream, evidence-based Western medicine? Everyone and his grandmother have had some form of knee surgery. Of course it works.

Hating to miss work, I plan on taking off only the day of surgery. Some of my colleagues question my judgment, while others reassure me that I will be running marathons within a week of surgery. My surgery is scheduled for 10 a.m. on a Wednesday. The preceding Monday, I receive a call from an anesthesiologist who takes my history and gives me some pre-operative instructions. I also receive a copy of these instructions in the mail. The instructions are straightforward: no aspirin or non-steroidal anti-inflammatories during the week prior to surgery, and no food or drink after midnight prior to the surgery.

I am a bad patient. Despite the very clear instructions directing me not to eat after midnight, I find myself in the kitchen at 2 a.m. on the morning of the surgery. What harm can be had by a cold piece of pizza and a handful of chips? I figure eight hours should be plenty of time for me to fully digest this early morning meal. Why do I do this? I hate being hungry, and I am afraid that if I don't eat something, I will have a crushing headache by noon. I keep my indiscretion to myself, since if I tell my wife, she may feel compelled to report me. I further transgress by drinking a cup of black coffee when I wake.

Beth drives me to the day surgery center at the main hospital. While waiting to be called back, I go to the bathroom a couple of times to urinate. Beth can tell I am nervous. Shortly thereafter, I am called back to the pre-operative holding room and given a gown. After gowning up, I sneak to a bathroom at least three more times. I hope to avoid needing a urinary foley catheter at all costs. Despite being a doctor, I am squeamish when it comes to having medical procedures performed on myself. It is embarrassment, as much as the pain, which I seek to avoid. I frequently tell Beth that when I am old and senile, she is to take me on an African safari, where I should be left out on the open plain to allow nature to run its course.

After a short eternity, Dr. J comes in to say hello and answer any lingering questions. There will be no foley! One indignity spared. He steps out, and a nurse comes in and preps me for surgery. She shaves my knee, starts an IV, and hangs a bag of intravenous fluids. She injects some anesthetic into my IV. The next thing I know the surgery is over, and I am being shaken awake by my wife. I feel a bit loopy, but good. After a short time in recovery, Beth is allowed to drive me home. The rest of the day is a blur. A few pain pills, a quiet room, maybe some dinner, and the next thing you know, I am getting up for work.

The day after surgery I feel pretty good. When I remove the post-operative ACE wrap, I note that my knee is swollen but aside from this, it looks fine. Over the ensuing week, the swelling gradually goes down, and I progress from limping to a fairly normal gait. I follow up with Dr. J to have the sutures removed, and he seems satisfied with my recovery. After one more week, the swelling has resolved and I feel 80% cured. I begin to ramp up my activity. My knee definitely is much better. I play basketball with my son in the driveway and even kick the soccer ball. No running, but otherwise I have my life back. The range of motion in my knee is still limited, and I get some soreness after a lot of activity, but I am not complaining. I am very satisfied with the outcome of the surgery until I make the mistake of talking on the phone with my friend Mark.

Mark is one of my oldest and dearest friends. He is a true physician-scientist. He performs cutting edge research at the University of Pittsburgh Medical Center. We have been best friends since high school in Gainesville, Florida. During our phone call, I mention my recent knee surgery, and Mark asks if I perhaps had a partial meniscectomy. I say, "Yes, I did." "Interesting," Mark replies, "I don't suppose you read the recent *New England Journal of Medicine* study that showed no benefit from that procedure?" I am flabbergasted. No, I had not read that article. I manage to excuse myself from the phone call, and I immediately jump online to Google "partial meniscectomy and the *New England Journal of Medicine*" (NEJM). I am stunned to find the publication Mark referred to, published in December of 2013.[1] It compared arthroscopic partial meniscectomy, the procedure I just had, with sham surgery. The sham group was the perfect placebo control group. The sham group went through the same procedural steps as the true surgical group, but in the sham group the arthroscope was inserted into the knee and the operator only touched the cartilage, rather than performing the surgery. The participants were blinded to which group they were a part of. The result was that there was no difference in outcomes between the two groups. My world is rocked. Instantly, I feel a throbbing in my knee. Goodbye placebo effect.

Over the next few weeks, I pay closer attention to the signals given off by my surgically repaired knee. I am forced to consider that the surgery may have been for naught. Despite this, I am hiking again and playing sports with my kids. My knee still has some pain, but it is clearly better. It is certainly not the knee of a twenty-year-old, but it is functional. Later, we finally receive the bills related to the surgery. Not cheap. The charge for the MRI of my knee was $1,073, but it was fully covered by my insurance. Hospital charges related to the surgery were $5,607, which was adjusted down to $3,622 by the insurance company, who paid 80%. The surgeon's bill was $2,550, adjusted down to $2,104, and again 80% covered by insurance. There was also a charge of $510 for "surgical assistance," and $920 for anesthesia. In the end, my portion for this surgery of questionable benefit was about $1,300.

When I delve further into the evidence to support meniscal surgery, I am forced to conclude that my choice to have surgery might not have been the wisest one. A second *NEJM* article, published in May of 2013, compared partial meniscectomy combined with physical therapy versus physical therapy alone. The patients had confirmed meniscal tears and evidence of mild-to-moderate osteoarthritis. The group that received physical therapy alone did just as well as the combined group.[2] I began to wonder if partial meniscectomy was even the best surgical option I could have entertained. According to a review by Scott Paxton and colleagues published in *The Journal of Arthroscopic and Related Surgery* in 2011, it was not.[3] Based on their review of the published literature, meniscal repair, basically suturing a torn meniscus back together, was superior to what I underwent, a partial meniscectomy.

I should have done my homework before "going under the knife." I foolishly believed that a commonly performed

“Western medicine” procedure, such as meniscal surgery, would be supported by well-founded research. Boy, was I wrong. This is a lesson learned. As I continue my exploration of alternative therapies, I will keep in mind that even “Western medicine” is often lacking in proof.

## Orthopedic Surgery

**Cost of initial consultation:** $100-$250

**Cost of follow-up visits:** $50-$250

**Cost of meniscal surgery:** Average cost nationally: $13,000 (range from $5,400-$36,700)[4]

**Covered by standard insurance policies:** Yes.

**Published research:**

Arthroscopic partial meniscectomy – The two best studies are as outlined above. Both were published in the *NEJM* in 2013, and both showed no benefit of partial meniscectomy over physical therapy alone.

There is lack of evidence supporting the management of several common orthopedic conditions. To the credit of the American Academy of Orthopedic Surgeons, they have begun to embrace evidence-based medicine and have a web-site with clinical practice guidelines and the current evidence supporting various practices.[5]

# Endnotes


1 Sihvonen, R., et al. Arthroscopic partial meniscectomy versus sham surgery for a degenerative meniscal tear. *N Engl J Med,* 2013;369(26):2515-24.

2 Katz, J.N., et al. Surgery versus physical therapy for a meniscal tear and osteoarthritis. *N Engl J Med,* 2013;368(18):1675-84.

3 Paxton, S.E., et al. Meniscal repair versus partial meniscectomy: a systematic review comparing reoperation rates and clinical outcomes. *J Arthroscopic and Related Surg,* 2011;27(9):1275-88.

4 http://newchoicehealth.com/directory/procedure/130/meniscectomy–searched on 6/4/2014

5 http://www.aaos.org/Research/guidelines/guide.asp

# Chapter 11 Give Me the Beet – Performance-Enhancing Drinks

Now that my knee is as good as new, I am ready to start biking seriously again. Running, on the other hand, is still not possible. If only there were a way to jump start getting into shape.

All athletes, whether they are professionals or weekend warriors like me, are searching for ways to improve their performance. We all want a silver bullet to rocket us to the podium or help achieve a new PR (personal record). Some choose to go the illegal route, while the rest of us sort through the many legal products claiming to give a leg up. It can be a challenge determining which claims are factual and which ones are pure fantasies. There is stiff competition among sports drinks to be recognized as "the one." Clearly, the selling of beverages can be lucrative; how else did Red Bull finance a leap from space? The question I have is … Do these drinks really work? Are the claims of enhanced performance mere bluster to part us from our hard-earned dollars? If you have purchased a Red Bull or Monster drink, you are aware they are not cheap. These drinks claim to help one run faster and longer and to be stronger, but how do I determine which one is the best? I will make it my quest to find out. After much contemplation, I devise the perfect experiment to determine which drink is really number one.

As part of my standard routine, I bike to work two to three days a week. One segment of my ride home is a steep 4.6 mile climb up the Blue Ridge Parkway. Periodically, I race up this segment of the ride while trying to best my prior times. More recently, I was introduced to a new application for mobile devices called STRAVA. Using the GPS technology in your phone, STRAVA tracks your route while recording your pace, time, and change in elevation. It also allows you to compare your time to other STRAVA users who have ridden the same route. Users designate specific segments of runs or bike routes that are particularly arduous and turn them into informal competitions. The person with the shortest time to complete any given segment is given the title King of the Mountain (KOM).

STRAVA is perfect for me. I yearn to see how I stack up against fellow cyclists, yet I fear the public ridicule of finishing last in a race. I have seen enough Asheville cyclists to know they are a serious lot. Recently, I was biking along the parkway when a peloton of riders overtook me. They were engaged in casual conversation with one another as they blew past me. They slowed down only briefly, gave me a once over, and then inquired if I perhaps was in the market for a new bike – the nerve. My bike may be twenty years old, but it was worth more than my car when I purchased it, and despite its age and mismatched parts I am deeply attached to it. I attempted to join the back of their pack only to be unceremoniously dumped within minutes. STRAVA is the app for me. It allows me to virtually race others while remaining semi-anonymous. I say "semi-anonymous" because your results are posted for others to see, but at least one is spared the sympathetic cheers that come with finishing near the back of a race. Cheers I know only too well.

It just so happens that the 4.6 mile segment of my ride home from work is popular among local STRAVA users. With the help of my oldest son, Connor, who recently turned 13, I form the following plan: I will pick several performance drinks and then compare their impact on my time trial performance on the 4.6-mile climb. STRAVA will record my times to ensure accuracy and allow me to see how I stack up against the rest of the local riders. My wife, Beth, will serve me the various drinks in the form of a smoothie along with standard ingredients (frozen berries, orange juice, and ice) in an attempt to keep me "blinded" from knowing what I am drinking. Only at the end of the experiment will I know which of the concoctions I drank. I will perform the segment under the influence of each drink and also once with no additive (the placebo). Today, a Saturday, I will time myself on the segment for the first time to establish a baseline.

As I glide down the mountain toward my workplace on a weekend, I begin to question the sanity of my plan. Do I really want to sacrifice precious weekend time riding the same segment of the parkway that I already cover several times a week? It would be nice to see some new scenery on the weekend. The experiment will only work if I perform my timed rides on the weekend when I am fully rested and not weakened by a hard day on the job. With these thoughts in mind, I reach the starting point at the bottom of the mountain. I pull up the STRAVA app on my iPhone and begin the ascent. The ride is a lot easier in the morning and without a backpack full of work materials. I push as hard as I can and complete the segment in 24 minutes, a personal best.

That evening, I reflect back on my morning's ride. It becomes clear to me that I can't go through with my original plan. Don't get me wrong; I am ecstatic with my performance. I set a new PR! Despite my euphoria, I cannot imagine racing up the same section of the mountain every weekend for the next six weeks – the same route I laboriously plod up two to three times a week, always at the end of a long workday. Beautiful as this part of the parkway may be, I have a hard time disassociating this weekend ride from my work routine. Weekends are weekends, and workdays are workdays. I would like to keep each in its separate compartment. As a result, I have drastically reconfigured my performance-enhancing drink (PED) experiment. The new plan is as follows:

Instead of repeating my workday climb, I will perform my weekly time trial on a different, even more popular STRAVA segment, referred to as the Elk Mountain TT (Time Trial). According to STRAVA, the Elk Mountain TT is a category 2 climb (1 is hardest and 5 is easiest). It is 4.8 miles in length and has a 5.3% average grade. There is a yearly race up Elk Mountain, which is part of the "Lung Buster Time Trial Series," so I presume it will not be easy.

Second, although I planned to compare various PEDs in a stepwise "blinded" fashion (using smoothies to mask the identity of the PED), I now doubt the feasibility of this plan. It is unlikely my wife can really blend such a great smoothie that I am unable to discern whether she added a can of Red Bull as opposed to a vegetable juice. Also, each PED comes with distinct instructions regarding the ideal time to drink it to maximize impact. Considering these barriers, I decide to strip my experiment of its last semblance to true science. Honestly, none of my other alternative medicine trials have been blinded so why should this be any different? Besides, whoever heard of a single-person, placebo-control study? Plus, by being aware of what I am drinking, I will be fully susceptible to the advertised claims promulgated by each product. Why should my experience differ from the Red Bull guy who parachuted from outer space? I will be able to fully describe my expectations that come with each PED, its taste, and the perceived effects it has on my performance.

Who are the contenders for best PED? Do any of them work? After exhaustive research (a fifteen-minute Internet search), I narrow the field to four drinks. Each claims to improve performance. I am referring to athletic performance, although a close source tells me at least one of these drinks may also improve another type of "performance" (hint – in the bedroom). The chosen drinks are Red Bull Energy, Gatorade G-series 01 Prime, Unbeetable, and coffee. Why these drinks? These are the only ones I can find claiming to enhance athletic performance. Coffee, the exception, is not marketed with this claim, but there has been more research regarding coffee's impact on athletic performance than the rest of the contenders combined.

First up is the ubiquitous Red Bull Energy Drink. According to the company's website, it will "give me wings." It is "fueled by a combination of caffeine, taurine, B-vitamins, sucrose, glucose, and alpine spring water." The website is a virtual Who's Who of professional athletes and daredevils who endorse Red Bull. Though I am not planning on jumping out of a spacecraft, I am looking forward to seeing what the Bull can do for me. Maybe I will find out it is all just a bunch of bull . . .

Contender number two for best PED is a relative new kid on the block, Unbeetable. Let me come clean right off the bat . . . I have a huge conflict of interest. One of my closest friends recently brought Unbeetable to market. Can I be more conflicted? Yes – I also hold a 1% stake in the company, and my wife is a salesperson. Will this bias me when I come to my analysis? Probably. Despite this conflict, I pledge not to fudge the results of my biking time trials, and I will attempt to remain truthful in my analyses. The scientist in me knows Unbeetable should not be included on this list, but the athlete in me cannot help but give it a try. Beetroot juice, the core ingredient of Unbeetable, is the rage in endurance sports. Any accomplished cyclist or runner is familiar with juicing beets. During the 2012 Summer Olympics, athletes used beetroot heavily. Why am I choosing Unbeetable and not a competitor beetroot drink? First, I have 3,000 bottles of Unbeetable in my garage; and second, I hate the taste of beets, but I am able to tolerate Unbeetable. There you have it, my full, heavily biased disclosure.

The third contender is Gatorade G-series 01 Prime. These drink names are getting complex. Whatever happened to plain old Gatorade? I grew up in Gainesville, Florida, and take pride in the fact that a local scientist invented Gatorade for the Florida Gators. Now they just call it G. What a crock. Despite this injustice, it is hard to leave G off the list. Of Gatorade's many performance drinks, only G-series 01 Prime is marketed to be taken prior to exercise to enhance performance. Go to the website and you can see the "science" behind the drink. I will give it a try. Go Gators!

Last, the universal pick-me-up, coffee. I must decide which java will fuel my performance – my standard home brew, Trader Joe's Dark, or Starbucks. I am not a Starbucks fan, so Trader Joe's Dark it is. Coffee is chock full of antioxidants, it purportedly boosts athletic performance, and it tastes good. Now that I have settled on the drinks . . . let the competition begin.

The following weekend, I race up Elk Mountain to establish my baseline. The beginning of this STRAVA segment starts about three miles from my front door. It is all downhill or flat from my doorstep to the starting point. When I arrive at the starting line, I am refreshed and ready to go. From the minute I leave Beaverdam Road and turn onto Elk Mountain Scenic Highway, I push myself as hard as possible. The climb is unrelenting, with steep grades and countless switchbacks. I am nearly spent when I come to a brief downhill segment, which leads into an open glade overlooking downtown Asheville. I relish the short reprieve before I start the final brutal ascent. The road is spray painted with exhortations left over from past races to "push it" and "almost there." One says, "You got this Moe." Who is Moe, I wonder? Finally, I reach the peak. It feels like I might have a cardiac arrest. Once my pulse has slowed, I pull my bike over to check out how I did on the Elk Mountain TT. My time is 33:47. I rank

314th of 461 participants. Not bad, but not in the top half as I had hoped. Of course, what was I expecting in a town of budding Olympians? I bet Lauren Tamayo, our local silver medalist, rides this segment several times a week, using a different STRAVA alias each time. I check out the KOM: it is Albert Pine in a time of 18:48. Are you kidding me? I was only at the halfway point when he was finishing. Perhaps Albert is an alias for Lance Armstrong. My initial ride has proven I have my work cut out for me. Maybe with the help of some "performance enhancement," I can crack the top half of the leaderboard by summer's end.

Another week passes, it is a crisp clear Saturday morning, and I am excited to try out the first contender for best PED on the market, Red Bull. The conditions are ripe for me to achieve a new personal best. I load myself with a healthy breakfast of cereal topped with fruit and a glass of orange juice. An hour later, I am raring to go. I pop open an 8–ounce can of Red Bull and quickly down the whole thing. It is my first Red Bull ever. I am pleasantly surprised. It has the color and consistency of ginger ale, is lightly carbonated, and has a slightly fruity taste. Not bad. I expected it to be dark, more akin to Coke or possibly Jolt cola, which was popular when I was in college. I remember my classmates drinking Jolt cola to fuel late-night drinking binges and also to stay awake during the inevitable all-night study sessions that followed. I have always perceived Red Bull to be the Jolt cola of the 21st century. I suppose I have been unfair.

Twenty minutes later, I am on my bike rolling down the road toward the Elk Mountain Time Trial start. I warm up my body and my legs by spinning my pedals at a rapid cadence while I glide down the three miles of road between my home and the starting point. It is a nice cool morning with the temperature in the sixties. Conditions are favorable. The Red Bull should be kicking in. Time to tame the mountain.

I turn on to Elk Mountain road and start the relentless climb. I choose not to wear a watch because I don't want to compare my splits with prior efforts. I plan on pushing myself as hard as I can go each time, and when I get home my STRAVA app will let me know how I did. After about five minutes, I feel pretty good. I am pushing a good steady pace. Often, I see black bears and wild turkeys along this stretch, but there is no wildlife along the road today to distract me. The pavement churns below me. I am a well-oiled machine. Aside from an occasional burp, undoubtedly due to the carbonation in Red Bull, I am doing fine. As I cruise into the open glade, which also happens to hold the most idyllic farmhouse with its own pond, I catch my breath and dig in for the final steep climb. I push through my pain on the final ascent and keep pumping until I reach the finish line. I then leisurely complete the rest of the ride home while basking in my accomplishment. Surely, I crushed the time from my baseline ride, and in doing so, set a new PR.

When I arrive home, I check my time for the Elk Mountain TT segment on STRAVA. I am flabbergasted to discover my time is 33:54. I actually went 7 seconds slower than the week prior. It appears I have been bucked off the Red Bull rather than riding it to victory. My ride felt so good. It is hard to conceive that not only was my time over a 4.8 mile course within 7 seconds of my prior ride, but that it was 7 seconds slower. Ouch. Not a ringing endorsement of Red Bull.

Next up in the competition for best PED is Unbeetable. A week has passed and once again, the conditions are ideal for me to have a good ride. It is a nice cool morning, and my body feels great. I twist open an 8-ounce bottle of Unbeetable and fill up my glass. Unbeetable is dark and foreboding with an eerie resemblance to blood. Fortunately, it does not have the classic smell of canned beets. I am not a beet lover, or even a beet liker. I take a sip. It is a bit too concentrated. I fill the remaining third of my glass with sparkling water. Much better. It is now quite drinkable. I ingest the whole drink in a few large gulps. I will begin my time trial in about two hours. Two to three hours is the suggested time to wait for maximum benefit.

Two hours later, I am at the base of Elk Mountain. Today, I hope to set a new PR. I also hope to move up in the STRAVA rankings. Perhaps I can even break into the top half of the standings. I begin the climb. I push myself hard throughout the whole ride. The pavement rolls by. On the final ascent, I am hyperventilating. Shaky, but undaunted, I reach the top. The ride felt good, but I felt good last week and ended up disappointed. I don't let my hopes get too high.

On arriving home, I check my recorded time on STRAVA: 32 minutes, 10 seconds. I crushed my prior times by over a minute and half! I set a new personal best, and my ranking in STRAVA for the Elk Mountain TT has risen from 314th place to 270th of 472 participants. Not quite in the top half, but I am making progress. I am pushing the envelope. Watch out Mr. King of the Mountain, here I come! On my rides home from work during the ensuing week, I feel strong. I am definitely making progress. I am sure I will be setting new PRs each Saturday from here on out. I eagerly anticipate the coming weekend.

The weekend is here again. Today is the ride I have been looking forward to the most: climbing Elk Mountain fueled by a double dose of java – Trader Joe's Dark to be exact. While PEDs such as Red Bull and Gatorade get all the hype, good old caffeine (I use this synonymously with coffee) has the data to support its role as a performance booster. Coffee is not only a great source of caffeine, but it is also brimming with anti-oxidants. In my estimation, man evolved with coffee. Coffee has been a staple of man's diet for hundreds of years. Undoubtedly, our bodies have adapted to maximize coffee's benefits. After all these years, the craving for coffee is surely imprinted in our genetic code. After enjoying a second large cup of my favorite steaming libation, I am ready to hit the hills. It is a nice cool morning, the sun is shining, and I feel great . . . until I start my ride.

Five minutes into the ride, I can tell I am in for a struggle. Where is my get up and go? I feel flat. I even have a bit of a headache. Jitteriness is understandable, but to be bereft of energy is hard to fathom. Maybe my ancestors were tea drinkers. Despite my sluggishness, I push myself to go as hard as possible, but I can tell that I am fighting a losing battle. Even the wild turkeys on the side of the road seem uninspired today. I keep waiting for an energy surge to kick in. Maybe a bear will pursue me. Alas, it is not to be. The entire ride is laborious. As I near the halfway point, a rider passes me so quickly I feel I am going backward. I attempt to keep him in my sights, but it is impossible on the curvy, climbing road. Even the open glade provides little respite. It is probably because I know what lies just beyond. When all hope seems lost, I finally tap into a hidden energy reserve and finish strong. Despite my finish, I am reluctant to see my final time.

35:12 . . . pitiful. My performance is one and a half minutes slower than my baseline effort and a full three minutes slower than my personal best. How can this be? I am well rested, and my legs feel strong (at least they did prior to the ride). I was well prepared, having done a couple of good rides during the week, and I had allowed myself the standard two days of rest. Maybe Trader Joe's Dark coffee is to blame. Maybe I should have chosen Starbucks.

My regular riding punctuated by my STRAVA challenge each weekend has gotten me in great shape, but I am starting to tire of the routine. I am ready to have my Saturdays back – I want to explore new venues. Finally I arrive at the end – the last time trial. After today, I do not think I can stomach riding up Elk Mountain again for a long while. Nevertheless, I feel strong; I should after five weeks of regular riding, culminating with an all-out race against the clock each weekend. Today, I am fueling my ride with the final contender in the best PED competition. Red Bull, Unbeetable, and coffee have all had their chance. Now it is Gatorade G-series Prime's opportunity to take the top spot, so I set out to buy some G-series Prime. You would think buying any Gatorade product would be a piece of cake. Gatorade has a ubiquitous presence on television, at sporting events, and in the supermarkets. Surprisingly, I have a hard time finding it on the store shelves. I check out our local supermarket – no drink. I run into a few convenience stores – no drink. Finally, I track it down at a big box sporting goods store. I suppose since it is so rare, they can charge a premium; sure enough, $2 for a 4-ounce packet.

Following the recommendations on the Gatorade website, I slurp down the whole packet twenty minutes before my planned ride. G-series Prime is composed of water, isomaltose, sugar, dextrose, maltodextrin, and vitamins B3, B5 and B6 – sounds yummy. It does not contain caffeine. After my weak rides on Red Bull and coffee, both drinks with high caffeine content, I am glad. The berry flavored G-Series Prime tastes like a syrupy version of the classic red Gatorade drink. Not bad. Its texture is a cross between a liquid and a gel.

Twenty minutes later, I attach my GoPro camera to my bike helmet to chronicle this final ride on Elk Mountain and start down my driveway. The GoPro is new to me. I hesitate using it. A GoPro video is the ultimate selfie. I let it sit in its box for the past six months until I finally had the gumption to figure out how it works. If you check out my video post of this ride, you will see I have not yet solved the GoPro riddle. A thunderstorm looms in the distance . . . perhaps this will be my GoPro's first and last ride; I am not sure the waterproof casing is on just right. Hopefully, filming with the GoPro and recording my ride on STRAVA have not exceeded my limited technological capabilities.

I turn onto Elk Mountain Scenic Highway and begin the time trial. I cruise up the first long incline with minimal suffering. Perhaps today is the day. I am a diehard Florida Gator fan, and I feel a strong allegiance to Gatorade, which was concocted by a University of Florida scientist to help the Florida Gator football team survive the heat. I will not be upset if a Gatorade product wins my competition; so much for my lack of bias.

Ten minutes into the ride, I feel strong until another biker blows by me. I try to keep pace with him, but in less than one minute, he is gone. Not a good omen. I push on. While cycling, I attempt to narrate key portions of the ride for my video, but I fear the audio will primarily be a sound tract of my gasping for air. Always on the lookout for nature, I again spot several wild turkeys, but they are not providing much entertainment today. I pass a three and half foot long black rat snake, which is attempting to cross the road. I look back to record its image, and nearly crash. Eyes back on the road for the final climb.

I ride hard all the way to the bitter end. My time is 33:44. No record today. This is the second fastest time I have posted while drinking the PEDs, but it is only three seconds faster than my non-enhanced baseline ride, and it is a good one and a half minutes slower than my personal best. No KOM awards for me. Albert Pine, your title is safe. This is not a knock on the G-series Prime drink. I like the taste and the fact that the recommended serving is only four ounces, but I can't say it did anything for me.

Well, there you have it: G-series Prime was the last of the PEDs to be tested. My personal trial has come to an end. Of the four performance drinks tested, Unbeetable is the clear victor. Of course, critics of my trial will point out that my highly unscientific study had only one participant – me. Plus, my experiment was heavily biased: I was aware of what I was drinking prior to each time trial, and I had every reason to want Unbeetable to be the winner (remember the 3,000 bottles in my garage). Despite this, I tried my best to give 100% effort each time up the mountain, regardless of which drink was being tested.

Now, I will change hats. Instead of being the guinea pig, I am the researcher. I comb the literature to research the science behind the claims of each drink. Why didn't I "grow wings" with Red Bull? How did 330 persons go faster than me up Elk Mountain if I really am Unbeetable? What is the proof any of these drinks work? My experiment certainly doesn't give the final answer to these questions.

A review of the ingredients of each drink reveals a few common themes. Caffeine is a major component of both Red Bull and coffee (80 mg in an 8.4 ounce can of Red Bull and 95 mg in a typical cup of coffee). Carbohydrates, primarily in the form of sugars, are present in large amounts in all four (Red Bull – 28 grams, Coffee – 8 grams per tablespoon of sugar, Unbeetable – 25 grams, and G1– 25 grams). Unbeetable is the only drink high in dietary nitrates. Beyond this, each drink has various other ingredients that may sound good, but for which there is no evidence that they enhance athletic performance: B-vitamins in Red Bull and G1, and anti-oxidants in coffee and Unbeetable.

I review each of the drink companies' websites to see what scientific justification they give to back up their claims. I then search Google and Pub Med (an online medical research library) to find more support for each drink or for the ingredients fueling the companies' claims. Caffeine, as an enhancer of sports performance, is well studied. Evidence shows caffeine improves performance in aerobic sports and, to a lesser extent, in high intensity (anaerobic) exercises such as cycling. Although the overall impact of caffeine remains inconclusive, the International Olympic Committee feels caffeine's influence is strong enough to require a limit on the amount of caffeine measurable in one's urine prior to competition. The impact of carbohydrates on performance is also well studied. The consensus is that carbohydrates, prior to endurance athletics such as cycling, improve performance. Nitrate, the active ingredient in Unbeetable, has scientific substantiation ranging from basic science research to clinical trials showing possible benefit in endurance sports. High nitrate consumption leads to blood vessel dilation and improved muscle efficacy.

Researching studies of the drinks themselves, rather than extrapolating benefits based on the ingredients, I find much less data. Red Bull is the best studied. I find three studies concluding that Red Bull improves aerobic and anaerobic performance. In one of these studies, participants improved their performance during a simulated cycling time trial after drinking Red Bull. I was unable to find any good studies evaluating coffee or G1's impact on athletic performance. Unbeetable has a study showing increased blood supply to parts of the brain in older persons, but no studies specifically looking at athletic performance. The supporting references on the Unbeetable website focus on the studies of dietary nitrates which is the main "active" ingredient.

How do I reconcile all this data? Caffeine, carbohydrates, and nitrates all have well substantiated benefits as enhancers of athletic performance. Hence, all of these drinks can rightly claim they "may" improve one's athletic performance. Red Bull has the most support with studies specifically evaluating its drink.

What will I drink prior to competition? I will probably stick with Unbeetable because it seems to work for me. The fact that I had my best ride after drinking Unbeetable will forever bias me. Plus, I am not a caffeine junkie. If you are afraid of getting fat, you should probably steer clear of all these drinks, with the exception of black coffee. All competitive athletes are looking to maximize results. PEDs appear to give them a slight edge. Each athlete will have to determine which PED works best for them.

## Performance-Enhancing Drinks

**Cost:** $2-$3/drink

**Published research:**

Red Bull – There are several small controlled studies showing improved endurance.[1,2]

Carbohydrates – Several studies support the benefits of carbohydrates (sugars) as beneficial for performance in endurance sports such as cycling.[3]

Caffeine – Well studied. Multiple studies confirm the benefit of caffeine on sports performance.[4]

Dietary Nitrates – Multiple studies ranging from basic research to clinical trials support benefits of dietary nitrates on athletic performance. The most obvious benefits appear during endurance sports, which require maximum exertion.[5,6]

# Endnotes


1 Ivy, J.L., et al. Improved cycling time-trial performance after ingestion of a caffeine energy drink. *Int J Sport Nutr Exerc Metab*, 2009 Feb:19(1):61-78.

2 Alford, C., et al. The effects of red bull energy drink on human performance and mood. *Amino Acids,* 2001:21(2): 139-50.

3 Smith, J.W., et al. Fuel selection and cycling endurance performance with ingestion of [13C]glucose: evidence for a carbohydrate dose response. *J Appl Physiol,* 2010 June;108(6):1520-9.

4 Burke, L.M. Caffeine and sports performance. *Appl Physiol Nutr Metab*, 2008 Dec;33(6):1319-34.

5 Lansley, K.E., et al. Acute dietary nitrate supplementation improves cycling time trial performance. *Med Sci Sports Exerc*, 2011 June;43(6):1125-31.

6 Larsen, F.J., et al. Dietary nitrate reduces maximal oxygen consumption while maintaining work performance in maximal exercise. *Free Radic Biol Med,* 201 Jan15;48(2):342-7.

# Chapter 12 Stroke It Like Derek Jeter – Titanium Necklaces

Have you ever wondered about those titanium necklaces worn by major league baseball players? Either the major leaguers are convinced the necklaces improve their performance, they are making a fashion statement, or the athletes are getting paid big bucks by the companies who make the necklaces. Not surprisingly, these necklaces are also the rage among Little Leaguers. Anything so pervasively adopted by the masses must be good. Am I missing out? Apparently the titanium imbues the necklace with special healing properties.

Recently, a good friend and his family visited from Ohio. His 13-year-old son, an avid baseball player, was wearing a titanium necklace. I decided this was a good time to learn more about the necklace and find out why he was wearing it. Carter said he hadn't had any injuries or joint pain since he began wearing it. Strange – I don't remember joint pain being a major issue as a child. Nevertheless, his endorsement piqued my interest. I search "titanium necklace" online and learn that titanium necklaces "balance the bioelectric current of the body and heighten its abilities." "It also has a healing ability that increases the condition of the body." Maybe this explains the long career of New York Yankee Derek Jeter. Despite being in his forties, he continues to pound out the hits. A titanium necklace sounds perfect for me. Since I turned 40 a few years back, my Yin and my Yang are out of whack. Maybe a titanium necklace will bring them back into equilibrium. I could certainly use some of those "special healing properties" for my aching knees, back, and shoulders. Perhaps if it fails to improve my pains, it will at least raise my batting average.

I make a trip to a local sporting goods store to purchase my very own titanium necklace. They can't be hard to find. Sure enough, hanging from the display near the check-out aisles are several varieties of titanium necklaces. They come in a wide range of colors and sizes and are endorsed by an impressive array of athletes. I choose a Phiten titanium necklace, the brand endorsed by baseball player Derek Jeter. I plunk down $40. Not cheap, but if it cures my aches, it will be worth every penny.

I am going to wear the necklace at all times for the next two weeks. Later that day, I slip on my titanium necklace and strut about the house displaying my new hardware. I feel kind of cool. Maybe I can reclaim my surfer roots. The last time I wore a necklace, I was in high school in Gainesville, Florida. Of course, wearing a gold chain and a tank top, or "muscle-T," in Florida was standard attire in the '80s. Although I am not self-conscious wearing the necklace around my family, I wonder if I will feel the same when in public. I am a well-respected doctor, or so I think. I don't want to impair my street cred.

Over the next week, while wearing the titanium necklace, I periodically assess the status of my aches and pains. On the evening of day number two, both of my knees ache after an intense game of roller hockey with my boys. I want to take some ibuprofen, but I decide against it. I will give the necklace a chance to work its magic. By day number seven of the titanium trial, my surgically repaired left knee is aching more than ever, my back is sore, and I still can't lie on my left side at night due to shoulder tendonitis. At the very least, I hoped my shoulder pain would improve. Heck, the necklace just about touches my shoulder; surely its healing powers should be able to emanate a few inches. In addition to the joint and muscle aches, my headaches have been acting up this week. Of course, lack of exercise due to daily rains and a deficit of sleep might also be to blame. I am at the midpoint of the titanium experiment, and so far I don't think the necklace is working. Perhaps the titanium has a delayed effect and week number two will be when I see the benefits.

Not only is the necklace not working wonders for my aches and pains, but I must admit that I feel a bit self-conscious when I am wearing the necklace in public. Normally I pride myself on not caring what others think – at least regarding my fashion sense, but with my necklace on, I feel like Don Johnson from the 1980s television show *Miami Vice*. I even think some of my friends are embarrassed to be seen with me. Perhaps unbuttoning my shirt down to my navel and exposing the necklace on my hairy chest while sitting with them in a restaurant has something to do with it. Despite my friends' look of repulsion, I do think the waitress is impressed.

While at an Asheville Tourists baseball game with my father, the necklace leads to a discussion regarding the benefits of titanium. My father, who has two titanium artificial hips, was heartened to learn of titanium's healing properties. He says he suffers from knee pain, back pain, and still has some stiffness in his hips. It seems that old age is taking its toll. "Thank goodness," he says, for the titanium in his artificial hips, since he can only imagine how bad things might be if the titanium wasn't working its magic.

As the two-week experiment comes to a close, my multitude of aches persists. In addition to the knee, back, and shoulder pain, I have a new pain in my calf from playing soccer. Despite the titanium necklace's failure to cure my pains, perhaps my hand-eye coordination has improved. There must be a good reason the major leaguers wear these necklaces. If it doesn't stop the pain, maybe it increases one's skills. I decide I should try my hand at batting practice.

I enlist two of my sons to join me at a nearby baseball diamond. My son David assumes the pitcher's mound to throw me a few pitches. As I step up to the plate while wearing my titanium necklace, I channel my inner Derek Jeter. I have laser focus, and my reflexes are heightened. My son throws the first pitch, and I take a mighty swing.

After 30 minutes of batting practice, I am forced to conclude that my baseball skills are no better. The titanium necklace is a bust. Am I surprised that the titanium necklace failed to live up to its billing? Not really. Despite claims that titanium can reduce pain by affecting the bioelectric current in the body, there is no scientific evidence to support this claim. Does the body have bioelectric currents? One might say so: our cells communicate with one another via an electrical current produced by chemically gated channels. Nerve cells are especially adept at rapidly transmitting electrochemical signals over long distances. Yet skin is a poor conductor of electricity, and there is no evidence that titanium has any influence on nerve conduction. Face the facts: If you buy yourself a titanium necklace, do it to be stylish, rather than to improve your health or batting average.

## Titanium necklaces

**Cost:** $10-$60

**Published research:**

There are no published randomized studies on titanium necklaces.

Numerous sites that sell titanium bracelets and necklaces claim pain reduction, healing, immune system boost, increased energy, and anti-inflammatory properties.[1]

# Endnote

1 www.livestrong.com/article/200694-the-benefits-of- titanium-bracelets

# Chapter 13 Adjusting my Polarity – Magnet Therapy

Titanium didn't do much for my "bioelectric current"; perhaps magnets will do a bit better. I don't understand the public's fascination with magnets. People sleep on magnetic mattresses, and they wear magnetic bracelets, necklaces, and back braces. Are they making a fashion statement, warding off evil spirits, or healing an injury? Talk to a believer and you will be regaled with a litany of theories of why and how magnets exert their benefit: "Our bodies are basically one big electric circuit." "The travel of nerve impulses and cellular communication require positively and negatively charged particles." "Even the iron in our blood carries a charge." It doesn't require a stretch of the imagination to see that magnets might have an impact on all of this polarized activity. Personally, I wonder if disrupting one's polarity is a good thing. I fear that magnets will screw up the well-worked-out equilibriums among all the protons, electrons, and muons in my body. Despite my reservations, proponents of magnet therapy don't seem concerned about throwing their electrical balances out of whack. Quite the opposite appears to be the case.

The purported health benefits of magnets are many. According to my online research, people have used magnets for thousands of years to treat various ailments, ranging from exercise-induced muscle soreness to schizophrenia. Although the exact mechanism by which magnets exert their healing influence remains poorly elucidated, many alternative practitioners eagerly embrace their healing potential. What type of magnets are we talking about – magnets holding up pictures of your loved ones on the fridge, or those used to lift the remains of a car? There are various types of magnets used for healing. The most widely used and freely available are "static magnets." They are called static because their magnetic field is constant. This contrasts with other magnets that use electricity to generate electrical impulses, such as those used for pulsed electromagnetic field therapy (PEMF), which as one might surmise, provides variable magnetic impulses and clearly is not static. These more advanced forms of magnet therapy generally require professional application. Being a do-it-yourselfer, I will start my investigation into the miracle of magnets with some store-bought static magnets.

My research reveals that several companies sell "static" magnets for home use. I log onto Amazon, my preferred shopping portal, and decide to buy two magnet arrays sold by Bioflex. Bioflex is the self-proclaimed "original magnet manufacturer" with magnets designed "specifically and exclusively for human and veterinary medical use." Wonderful – if they don't work for me, I can use them to heal my dog. The Bioflex website claims its concentric circle magnets are able to modulate the body's normal production of anti-inflammatory chemicals within affected tissues and thereby promote pain relief. It sounds like just what my sore back needs. Despite my well-chronicled visits to multiple health practitioners, I continue to suffer from chronic lower back pain, periodic headaches, and insomnia. With these ailments in mind, I order the Bioflex Deluxe Lumbar Back Support and the Bioflex Magnetic Head Band for $59.99 and $29.99 respectively. My plan is to wear both of these as much as possible during the next four weeks. I can wear the back brace, which is embedded with the static concentric magnets, at all times. I should be able to conceal it under my clothing. I will wear the head band while I sleep at night. Needless to say, I will keep away from the MRI machines at the hospital and avoid curious children carrying paperclips and needles.

A week has passed; I am honoring my commitment to wear the back brace at all times. Aside from having embedded magnets, it looks and feels like any other Velcro back brace. Perhaps it is a bit thicker, but that is the only difference I can appreciate. Overall, I don't mind wearing the magnets except for the heat the elastic bands create. At baseline, I am already prone to sweating. If you put a thick back brace and elastic head band on me, I turn into a fountain of sweat. I frequently wake up at night drenched in a pool of perspiration.

I decide to take my magnet wearing to the next level. Despite some misgivings, I decide to wear both the back brace and magnetic head band to work. The medical staff isn't able to take me seriously; they break into large smiles when I enter the room and degenerate into full-scale laughter as I leave. On top of this, my patients are not so eager to be treated by a doctor who wears a head band. This seems discriminatory to me. No one complained when LeBron James wore a headband. Why should I be treated any differently? After a couple of days, despite my desire to stand up for the rights of head band wearers everywhere, I am compelled to stop wearing the head band to work; my patients have been canceling their future appointments. Nevertheless, I continue to wear the back brace at virtually all times, and I wear the head band while in the privacy of my own office and while sleeping at night. My wife is used to my antics and barely bats an eye when I crawl into bed wearing both my magnetic back brace and head band.

I continue doing my regular activities of biking, tennis, and kayaking while taking frequent note of how my back is feeling, whether I am more or less headachy, and if I am sleeping well. I will be satisfied with the magnets if I see improvement in just one of these areas. The one activity I put on hold is backwoods hiking, since I worry about the impact of the magnets on my compass. I imagine being lost deep in the Smoky Mountains with the needle of my compass twirling around uncontrollably as I blindly search for civilization.

The weeks fly by during my experiment. Perhaps I should have reserved this evaluation until the cooler months of the year. Our electricity bill will undoubtedly be much higher than usual this month – I have dialed the thermostat lower and lower each evening in hopes of staving off the inevitable sweats generated by being ensconced in magnets. Also, I have developed a beautiful skin rash on my back and abdomen due to the persistently wet, warm environment created by the back brace. I am a fungus breeding ground. Enough of my complaints; the one question you are asking is . . . Do the magnets work? Are my back pain and headaches gone? Am I sleeping peacefully through the night?

Unfortunately, the answer is "no." My back aches more than ever. It now also itches due to the rash. My headaches have not changed. In truth, they may be a bit worse. The constriction of the elastic head band seems to exacerbate my headaches. Last, unsurprisingly, my insomnia has only worsened. After four weeks of wearing these magnets, I am ready to cast them off. Not only have my maladies persisted, but I am also $90 poorer (the cost of the magnets). Also, my wife thinks I am a leper due to my extensive rash. Others may have found relief from "static magnets," but not me. It is time to seek professional help.

What type of professional help you might ask? No more wimpy store-bought contraptions for me. It is time to try pulsed electromagnetic therapy (PEMF). It sounds like something from *Star Trek*. "Set phasers to stun – the Klingons are energizing their pulsed electromagnetics." You get the picture. According to *Alternative Medicine Guide – The Definitive Guide*, researcher Albert Davis, while investigating the impact of magnets on animals, found that magnets could kill cancer cells and be used to treat arthritis, glaucoma, and infertility. A Dr. Wolfgang Ludwig said magnetic field therapy can be used to "treat every organ without chemical side effects." Sign me up.

I Google "pulsed electromagnetic field therapy, Cleveland, OH," the city where I started my alternative medicine journey. I find a few references to various articles, but no links to local practitioners. When I repeat the search and substitute "Asheville, NC" for "Cleveland, OH," I find several practitioners who practice PEMF. I love this town. As I delve deeper, I locate two practitioners not far from my home that perform PEMF using a MG-33 device. I am not sure what this means, but I am eager to find out. I select the office closest to home and arrange an appointment.

A few days later, I escape from work during my lunch hour. The term "lunch hour" is a misnomer. Usually, I scarf down a sandwich while writing patient notes in my office. The sheer volume of crumbs lodged in my keyboard attests to this practice. I arrive at the clinic, which provides "integrated health solutions." It is located in a renovated two-story house. As I open the office door, the aroma of burning incense greets me. Sitting at a computer near the entrance is the doctor I have come to see. She asks if I am Scott; I say, "Yes." She then leads me directly to a small room with an easy chair in the corner. She is a very pleasant woman. She is gentle in nature and has a soothing voice. She deposits me in the easy chair and pulls up another chair opposite me. "What brings you here?" she asks. I tell her my left knee bothers me despite having had arthroscopic knee surgery six months ago. I also mention that I suffer from chronic lower back pain, but I make it clear that today I want to focus on the knee. She agrees. It doesn't take me long to realize she is a true believer. She herself had a "creaky" knee, which improved markedly with just one PEMF treatment. She had been at an "alternative medicine" trade show, and a man convinced her to try out the display MG-33 on her own knee. Immediately after the treatment, she had increased flexibility and decreased pain in her knee, and it has not recurred. It was this positive experience that led her to purchase the device for her practice. She says perhaps her knee problem may not have been as bad as mine; she had never had surgery on hers, but despite this, she thinks a single treatment, or at most a few treatments, should do the trick.

I glance at the MG-33 device, which sits on the floor next to my easy chair. It looks like a guitar amplifier. Hanging on the wall next to me are several circular clear tubes with wires running through them. They look like contraptions Dr. Frankenstein might use to raise the dead. Apparently, these coils of wires plug into the MG-33. I become a bit nervous, but I choose not to express my growing concern. It is hard not to trust this gentle woman, who also practices acupuncture and naturopathy.

The doctor hands me some forms to fill out and steps out of the room. These include the standard health history forms, next of kin, and the like. Also included is a disclaimer regarding PEMF therapy and an information sheet about the MG-33. The disclaimer states that PEMF is "not understood by allopathic medicine" and the MG-33 device is not FDA approved and makes no claims of cure. Not a ringing endorsement. The one-page informational sheet about the MG-33 explains that all persons will benefit from its use. It then goes on to explain how the treatment is done and what to expect. Hook me up. I am ready for my "total body energetic recharge."

While waiting for the doctor to return, I again inspect the multiple electrical coils hanging on the wall. I hope the doctor knows what she is doing. I notice there is also a detoxifying foot bath on the floor. I will be sure to avoid the footbath while plugged in. Just as my nervousness nears a crescendo, the doctor returns. Time to get down to business. She had instructed me to stay fully clothed. Apparently, my clothes won't have any impact on the MG-33. She selects a coil and proceeds to plug one end of it into the MG-33. I am instructed to pass the circular coil over my head and slowly down my upper body until I reach my waist. She turns a knob, which causes the coil to emit a tapping sound similar to two marbles being knocked together. She turns up the electrical current until I can feel the tapping. As I move the coil down my body, I can feel a pulsation and, with it, my muscles begin contracting. She says this part of the procedure is diagnostic rather than therapeutic. "Sites of cellular damage and injury will feel discomfort." As I pass the coil down my body, I also get the sensation that my internal organs are fluttering. When I get to the level where the coil encircles my waist and groin, I feel a mild pain in my right groin, a site where I think I have a small hernia. She has me sit back in the chair with the coil around my waist. My organ fluttering continues. Not painful, yet not really comfortable. After about ten minutes, she says it is time to focus on my knee.

She has me remove the large coil and in its place she attaches two smaller electrical coils, which are held together by a Velcro strap and placed over my left knee. She dials up the current until I again feel the tapping sensation. She adjusts it until I appreciate the vibration, but not to the point that it elicits pain. She sets the timer for 20 minutes and steps out of the room. I kick back in the chair and read the newspaper. This sure is a lot less hassle than physical therapy. If this does the trick, I may never stretch again.

I finish the newspaper and begin to feel antsy. Normally, I would be scrolling through the email on my iPhone, but the doctor explicitly told me to keep my credit cards and electronics at least five feet away from the magnetic coils. My

PEMF treatment will be much more costly if it forces me to buy a new phone. As the 20 minutes is nearing its end, I am unable to contain myself any longer. With the coils still firmly attached to my left leg, I hop across the room and grab my iPhone off the counter. I keep the arm holding my iPhone outstretched while I hop back to the recliner. My phone is still working so I take a selfie with the MG-33 coils wrapped around my leg. I hop the phone back to the safety of the far counter. Shortly thereafter, the MG-33 clicks off. I get up, remove the coils, and do a few deep knee bends. Amazingly, my knee feels pretty good.

I walk out to the waiting room, where the doctor is sitting. She prints out my bill. The bill comes to a mere $20 – one dollar for each minute of PEMF therapy on my knee. What a bargain. This is cheaper than either the titanium necklace or the static magnets. I just received one hour of professional consultation and treatment, and my bill is only $20. There must be a catch. I wait for the doctor to tell me about the need for repeated therapies of increased duration (and cost). But no, when I ask about return visits, she says, "Only if you feel you need it." This woman obviously would have failed out of business school. She says I can come back in a few weeks if my knee starts bothering me again, but she is hopeful that the one treatment will be all I need. I walk outside into the sunlight with a smile on my face.

My knee feels pretty good. When I get back to the hospital and climb four flights of stairs to my office, I notice a dull ache returning to my inner knee. I assume all the benefits of the MG-33 have vanished, but surprisingly, it is not the case. My knee actually feels much better than normal over the ensuing two weeks despite doing the activities that usually aggravate the knee – tennis with my son and hiking in the mountains. I intended to return for a second treatment to do more "research" on the process, but my knee feels too good to justify a return. PEMF seems to have done wonders for my knee. Perhaps my improvement is merely psychological – the placebo effect working its magic, or maybe I am just at a good point in the random fluctuations in my knee pain. Whatever the reason, I am now curious about the other treatments offered by the doctor. Perhaps the ionic detox footbath will help my headaches.

## Magnet Therapy

**Cost of static magnets:** $20-$100

**Cost of Pulsed Electromagnetic Therapy (PEMF):** $20-$50 session

**Covered by standard insurance policies:** No

**Published research:**

Static Magnets:

**How do they work?** Original claims that static magnets affect local blood circulation have been disproved.[1] There is weak evidence that static magnets may affect muscle metabolism[2], but this falls far short of an explanation of how they work – if they do at all.

There are many small non-randomized studies from which one can make limited inferences. Several of these small studies suggest benefit for rheumatoid arthritis, peripheral neuropathy, post-surgical pain, musculoskeletal pain.[3] Among more familiar peer reviewed journals, one study found benefit of magnetic bracelets for osteoarthritis pain of the hip and knee,[4] while a study using static magnets for chronic low back pain did not show benefit.[5] The National Center for Complementary and Integrative Health website states that "scientific evidence does not support the use of magnets for pain relief."[6]

Pulsed Electromagnetic Field Therapy:

**How do they work?** Again, how they work is murky. The belief is that PEMF stimulates cellular repair by stimulating the electrical and chemical processes in injured tissue. How it actually does this is anybody's guess.

Several small studies have found benefit from PEMF for osteoarthritis, urinary incontinence, multiple sclerosis, erectile dysfunction, migraines, and postoperative pain. I found further support for PEMF for knee arthritis[7] and pain management after oral surgery. On the flip side, I found studies that showed no benefit for knee arthritis[8] and no benefit for migraines.

Detoxifying foot baths:

By all measures, these are a scam. The premise is that when feet are placed in the foot bath, an electrical current will draw out the toxins from your body. There is no physiological basis for this claim, and when studied, there is no evidence of decreased toxic elements in one's body.[9] The water does change color due to the electrolytic corrosion of the metal electrodes, and it is soothing, as placing one's feet in hot water usually is, but it does not remove toxins.

# Endnotes


1 Martel, G.F., Andrews, S.C., Roeboom, C.G. Comparison of static and placebo magnets on resting forearm blood flow in young, healthy men. *J Orthop Sports Phys Ther,* 2002;32:518-524.

2 Engstrom, S., Markow, M.S., McLean, M.J., et al. Effects of non-uniform static magnetic fields on the rate of myosin phosphorylation. *Bioelectromagnetics*, 2002;23:475-479.

3 http://healthlibrary.epnet.com/GetContent.aspx?token=e0498803-7f62-4563-8d47-5fe33da65dd4&chunkiid=33778

4 Harlow, T., et al. Randomised controlled trial of magnetic bracelets for relieving pain in osteoarthritis of the hip and knee. *BMJ,* 2004 Dec 18;329(7480):1450-4.

5 Collacott EA, et al. Bipolar Permanent Magnets for Treatment of Chronic Low Back Pain-A Pilot Study. *JAMA,* 2000 Mar 8:283(10):1322.

6 https://nccih.nih.gov/health/magnet/magnetsforpain.htm.

7 Ryang, W.S., et al. Effects of pulsed electromagnetic field on knee osteoarthritis: a systematic review. *Rheumatology (Oxford),* 2013 May;52(5):815-24.

8 Ozguclu, E., et al. Additional effect of pulsed electromagnetic field therapy on knee osteoarthritis treatment: a randomized, placebo-controlled study. *Clin Rheumatol*, 2010 Aug:29(8):927-31

9 Kennedy, D.A., et al. Objective assessment of an ionic footbath (IonCleanse): testing its ability to remove potentially toxic elements from the body. *J of Environ and Pub Health*, 2012, 1-13.

# Chapter 14 You Are Becoming Very Sleepy – Hypnosis

I spent the past several months attempting to remedy my many physical complaints. Now it is time to tackle my greatest infirmity – my mind. I am not keen on electroshock therapy or undergoing a lobotomy, but I am intrigued by hypnosis. I always doubted I could be hypnotized. My wife frequently points out that I am a Capricorn, astrologically symbolized as a goat. Apparently, goats tend to be practical, evidence based, and always skeptical. Any reference to astrology elicits an eye roll from me – evidence substantiating her point. I admit I am innately skeptical of anything "spiritual" or requiring faith. Needless to say, I do not regularly attend church. There are similarities between some alternative therapies and religion. Both require openness to ideas that might initially seem counterintuitive and also a willingness to be healed. I struggle with blind faith: I want to know why things are the way they are. We were born with incredibly complex minds; shouldn't we be using them? "Just believe" is a hard pill for me to swallow.

Last week, my wife's college roommate and her family spent a night at our house on their way to Alabama. Both she and her husband are close friends and wonderful conversationalists. At some point, the discussion turned to my explorations of alternative medicine and the next experience on my ledger: hypnotherapy. David regaled me with his experiences being hypnotized. He recounted one episode at a local bar where my wife and his future spouse, Christina, were also present. He and several others were chosen out of the audience to be hypnotized on stage. The hypnotist gauged that David was among the more receptive candidates to hypnotic suggestion and singled him out for additional instructions. While still on stage, the hypnotist had David fill his pockets with napkins. Then the hypnotist planted the suggestion that once David returned to his seat and sat down, he would feel the napkins burning his legs, and he would jump up and exclaim a particular phrase. After a few more demonstrations by the hypnotist, he awakened the group from their hypnotic state, and David returned to his seat. Upon sitting down, he immediately leapt to his feet and exclaimed, "I am Tarzan, King of the Monkeys" as he frantically tore the burning napkins from his pockets. David had clearly been hypnotized. Hearing this story made me wonder if I too can be hypnotized.

David will be the first to admit he is very receptive to otherworldly ideas. His astrologic sign is Gemini, same as my wife, which they both claim makes them more spiritual and open to new ideas. "Baaahh," I say – the goat in me has spoken. These Geminis are stirring up my competitive juices. Goat or not, now I really want to be hypnotized. I may have been resistant to hypnotism three years ago, but I think it might work now. My alternative medicine experiences opened my eyes. I am a changed man; I am much more receptive to new approaches than I was at the beginning of my alternative medicine journey. I decide it is time to book an appointment with a hypnotist.

There are a plethora of hypnotists in Asheville. How will I choose one? Groupon, of course. I am an avid fan of Groupon. Who knew there were so many things I needed and all at half price? Groupon has a half-price deal for two hypnotherapy sessions with a CD to boot. I check out the doctor's web page, and I am impressed. The doctor not only has a PhD, but a whole bunch of other letters in her title. She even has a friendly picture of her and her horse. What more can

I ask for? Her website lists common problems treated with hypnosis and supporting scientific literature for the claims.

Anxiety and insomnia are the reasons I seek help (as well as the general desire to see if I can be hypnotized). The past several weeks have been very stressful. Work has been busy, and I have been racing against several looming deadlines. As a result, I feel like I have a hole in the pit of my stomach, and I have not been sleeping well. Unlike my past bouts of insomnia when my primary challenge was falling asleep, I am now waking up throughout the night and having difficulty falling back asleep. My Type A personality has clicked into overdrive. Every time I awaken, I rehash the same list of things that I need to get done at work. I am turning into a sleep-deprived bundle of nerves. I am eager to see if hypnotherapy can work for me. I purchase the Groupon and schedule an appointment.

Before I know it, the visit is upon me – time to get hypnotized. As suggested by her website, this hypnotist is no ordinary hypnotist. She has a PhD in neurosciences and a bevy of other degrees. With such lofty titles, I expect her office to be in a large hospital with an attached laboratory filled with ominous-appearing contraptions with wires and sensors for measuring brain activity. This is not the case. Her office is not located in a large medical complex; instead, it is in the back of a yoga studio. It takes me a while to find her office – I was not expecting it to be in a yoga studio. Finally, after ascertaining I am in fact in the right place, I take a seat by the yoga check-in desk while awaiting the doctor's arrival. I feel out of place in my tie and work clothes. While I wait for the doctor, scantily clad yogis file by for their noon yoga session. The doctor arrives ten minutes late, reportedly having been caught up in Asheville's notorious noon rush hour. I say this tongue in cheek because Asheville has almost no traffic, part of the reason I love this town.

My first impression of the doctor is that she is not a stereotypical neuroscientist. Instead of a white doctor's coat, she wears a stylish tight dress and has short, cropped, dyed-black hair – think Joan Jett. She is lithe, muscled, and adorned with numerous tattoos exposed along the margins of her dress. She ushers me into her office, which is small and spartan in appearance. The walls are bare, and a 1940s chaise lounge is the prominent feature of the room. Soothing music plays softly in the background. The doctor motions for me to take my place on the chaise lounge while she sits down in an upright chair positioned at the lounge's head, assuming the classic psychiatrist-patient position.

The doctor asks what I hope to gain from hypnotherapy. I mention my Type A personality, feelings of stress related to work, and difficulty sleeping. "How do you relax?" she asks. "By exercising, having a beer after work, and chilling out while watching Netflix with my wife after the kids have gone to bed," I reply. She asks me to describe my image of total relaxation. "Lying on the beach with a margarita in my hand," I respond. She smiles. The doctor then gives me some relaxation exercises I should perform several times each day to briefly escape from the multiple demands placed on me and to clear my mind. Basically, it is a 30-second exercise with three steps: first, one takes in all visual stimuli while focusing on none individually; second, one takes in all auditory stimuli while focusing on none individually; and third, one takes in all tactile stimuli while focusing on none individually. She says this is a quick way to briefly decompress, even in the midst of a busy workday. This is not a great exercise to do while driving. Shifting gears back to the upcoming hypnosis session, she asks me to choose a trigger that will tell my body it is time to enter full relaxation. She says I should pick something I do every night before I go to bed. I choose the act of closing my book at night before I go to sleep.

We begin the hypnotherapy session. In the classic Hollywood depiction of hypnotism, the psychiatrist guides the patient into a deep sleep-like trance and is able to delve into his innermost secrets. Upon awakening, the patient remembers none of the session. The doctor states she is very capable of doing just that, but it is not the goal of today's session. I will remember everything. I am a bit disappointed. She asks me to let go of my inhibitions and relax. I lie back in the chaise lounge and close my eyes. She has me focus on relaxing my muscles in a stepwise fashion from the top of my head down to the tips of my toes. I wonder if I will fall asleep. In a soothing voice, she leads me down a flight of ten stairs with an open door at the bottom leading to a beach. With each step downward, she instructs me to double my relaxation. Eventually, I make it to a tranquil beach where I lie in the sand with a margarita nearby. She tells my worries to leave me in little bubbles that rise above me and then float away like clouds on a gentle breeze. The sand is warm, and I have no cares. After relaxing for several minutes on the beach, she instructs me to visualize a candle. The flame is warm with an aura surrounding it. As I stare into the flame, she guides me into an empty blackness. I feel it. My mind is blank. She says I will achieve this state of total relaxation each evening when I close my book and place it on my bedside table. She continues to reinforce that I am totally relaxed and free of worries. After a while, she says she will count to three, and with each count I will be closer to awakening, and on three I will open my eyes. I am so relaxed I am unsure I will be able to open my eyes. Somehow, I force my eyes to open on three. I feel a bit stunned and very relaxed. She gives me a warm smile and asks how I feel. "Relaxed," I say. She stands up and moves to the other side of the room to sit behind her desk. The session has come to an end.

I rise from the chaise lounge and sheepishly pull out my Groupon and hand it to her. We schedule a second session, and she gives me a CD, which I am to listen to on my own. She also reminds me to practice "zoning out" as she instructed. As I drive back to work, I am completely relaxed. I don't turn on the radio for fear of losing my Zen state. I contemplate whether or not I have been hypnotized. I am not sure. What does it mean to be hypnotized? I am definitely relaxed. I am eager to try the techniques she has shown me and to listen to her CD. Will I fall instantly into a state of relaxation each night when I close my book?

During the next two weeks, I do my best to follow her recommendations. Twice a day, I attempt to "zone out" for a minute. During this time, in accordance with her instructions, I observe all visual stimuli, all noises, and all sensations while focusing on none. It is not a difficult exercise, and over the course of the first week, I get better and better at it. I am not sure this exercise noticeably decreases my stress level, but it does force me to take a break from my busy to-do list each day. Also, on at least two occasions before going to sleep, I listen to the CD for "Anxiety Release" given to me by the hypnotist. The CD is a form of guided hypnosis and is very similar in content to the hypnosis session I had in the office. The one drawback to the CD is that it takes a good 20 minutes. I find myself struggling to keep awake so that I can complete the session. Do I become hypnotized during these sessions? I am not sure.

During my hypnosis session with the doctor, she suggested I would assume a state of deep relaxation triggered by closing my book each night. This trigger has been quite effective. I do not know why it works, but I feel an overwhelming sense of relaxation upon closing my book, and I fall asleep quickly. In fact, I am wary of reading my book during the day for fear I will be overcome with a desire to sleep when I close the book. Fortunately, the majority of my reading during daylight hours consists of online articles, magazines, and newspapers. I foresee myself reading a chapter from my book at lunchtime and then waking up several hours later to find it is evening, and I have skipped an afternoon of seeing patients – kind of a modern day Rip Van Winkle. I doubt my boss or my patients would be appreciative.

My dalliance with hypnosis has piqued my interest in the entire field of hypnotherapy. The idea of tapping into one's subconscious to affect change in one's daily life is fascinating. I need to know more. I seek more information from my father-in-law, Dr. T.S. Kim, a retired psychiatrist. T.S. is one of the kindest, gentlest, and wisest men I have encountered. I don't tell my wife, but the real reason I married her was to have T.S. be my father-in-law. The one catch to seeking T.S.'s counsel is that at 87 years old, he is very hard of hearing. Rather than struggle to comprehend conversation, T.S. now favors recounting his prior experiences, particularly his Korean War experiences, which are fascinating and usually able to keep me enthralled for hours, but not my current topic of interest.

During our most recent visit to Hickory, North Carolina, I pull up a chair next to T.S. and ask him to tell me how he used hypnosis when he practiced psychiatry. After a few misunderstandings (first, his thinking I have asked about the Carolina Panthers and then perhaps the ongoing conflict in the Ukraine), I get him to address his views on hypnotism. He says, "Yes, hypnotism can be very effective. I incorporated hypnotism into my practice with good results. I have a few books I can give you on the subject." Then, apparently done with the topic of hypnosis, he begins regaling me with a familiar tale of his youth in North Korea during the times of Japanese occupation. It appears this is all T.S. will tell me about hypnotism today. At the end of our visit, T.S. gives me a couple of circa 1950 books on hypnotism.

On arriving home, I take a look at the books T.S. has given me. *Hypnotism* by G.H. Estabrooks, "one of American's leading psychologists," according to the book jacket, must have created quite a stir when it was published. Dr. Estabrooks contends people can be hypnotized against their own will. His book reviews hypnotic techniques and discusses the use of hypnosis, not only for medical conditions, but also for its possible use to perpetuate crime and as a tool of warfare. Imagine hypnotizing a legion of soldiers to do your bidding without concern for their own wellbeing. Surely, Vladamir Putin is using this trick on his military. The second book, *The Nature of Hypnosis*, takes a more Freudian approach. Its author, Dr. Paul Schilder, observes "hypnosis is also rooted in sexuality." My favorite quote from Dr. Schilder's work is, "Hypnosis represents the pleasure of surrender." I think Dr. Schilder may have hit upon the truth. One needs to surrender, putting skepticism aside, to experience the benefits of hypnosis. This has become my goal. I strive to fully open my mind so that I can delve into my own subconscious. More than ever, I strive to be hypnotized. I have made progress in the past two weeks, but I have much further to go. I have experienced moments of serene calm I have rarely experienced before. Unfortunately, these moments have been fleeting. In the coming weeks, I will attempt to lower the barriers I have erected around my subconscious in an effort to realize the full benefits of hypnotherapy.

Today is my second visit with the hypnotist. After two weeks of research into the principles of hypnosis and my subsequent attempts to apply this newly found knowledge, I have a host of questions to ask my hypnotist. I am eager to harness the untapped potential of my subconscious. Despite my eagerness, I have the nagging feeling I am coming up short. Up to this point, I am not sure I have been successfully hypnotized. The more I read and the more I experiment with guided hypnosis, the more confused I am regarding what hypnosis really means. This is one visit I am really looking forward to.

When I arrive at the yoga studio, the receptionist immediately leads me to the hypnotherapy room. The hypnotist sits in the upright chair at the head of the chaise lounge. She welcomes me and motions for me to take my place on the chaise. After a few pleasantries, I eagerly relate the events of the past two weeks. I then launch into my list of questions. Foremost among the questions are: "How do I know if I am being successfully hypnotized?" and "What evidence is there that hypnotism really works?" I hope I don't offend her. She smiles knowingly. Apparently, I am not the first to express these doubts. She reminds me that she too has a strong scientific background; in fact, she spends the majority of her day synthesizing neuropeptides for clinical and basic science research. She also refers me to her website, which gives examples of clinical studies substantiating the benefits of hypnotherapy.

She explains that humans, on average, only utilize 12% of their brains.* Hypnosis attempts to access a much larger portion of the brain via the subconscious. She also relates two anecdotes to illustrate the potential power of hypnosis. The first has to do with her multiple tattoos, which I commented on previously. She confides that getting a large tattoo can be extremely painful. I nod in agreement (as if I have multiple tats hiding under my shirt). She says when she got her first tattoos, she had to take multiple breaks during their application due to intolerable pain. Now, with the aid of self-hypnosis, she sleeps while getting tattoos. I look

* The myth that we use only 10% of our brain has been attributed to Albert Einstein, who used this statement to explain his towering intellect. This myth is just that, a myth. Brain researchers using imaging technology have shown that most of the brain's regions are continually active and that over a day you use 100% of your brain.[1]

at her incredulously. "But how do I know if I am capable of being hypnotized?" I ask.

She then tells me of a patient, similar to myself, who derived benefit from the hypnosis sessions, but was unsure whether she was truly being hypnotized. By mutual consent, during the subsequent hypnosis session, the hypnotist placed a subconscious trigger to confirm to the patient she had indeed been hypnotized. The hypnotist planted the suggestion that anytime the patient saw the color green, she would feel warm and happy. When the patient returned for the next visit, she was ecstatic. She claimed to have never been as happy as when she was sitting at a stoplight and witnessed it turning green. I am impressed. Am I being fooled? Perhaps, but the hypnotist strikes me as very professional and not prone to hyperbole.

Now I am more excited than ever by the possibilities of hypnotism, and I am ready to begin my second hypnosis session. The hypnotist concocted a new guide specifically for insomnia, one of my original complaints. I lie back in the chaise and close my eyes. While background music gently plays, the hypnotist has me focus on my breathing and then leads me through progressive relaxation of all my muscle groups. She counts backward from ten, and I find myself on a grassy knoll overlooking an idyllic beach. I am holding a balloon in my hand, which contains all my daily demands and worries. I release the balloon, and it slowly floats over the horizon and out of sight. She then leads me down the grassy hill to a bed lying in the shade of a stand of trees along the beach's edge. I lie down in the bed, which is incredibly comfortable. Feeling relaxed and carefree, I am instructed to visualize the dancing flame of a candle. I stare into the flame. The hypnotist implores me to sleep soundly throughout each night, unperturbed by background noise, and if I am awakened, I will be able to promptly fall back to sleep.

She mentions tapping into my subconscious mind and gives other instructions that I am unable to recall. She then counts backward from three, and I am awake.

Similar to my first session, I feel very relaxed. I struggle to stand up and reorient myself to the wakened world. I stumble out of the office. Once again, as I drive back to work, I reflect on the hypnosis session. I feel like I am on the cusp of being hypnotized, but have not yet reached nirvana. Perhaps hypnosis is just a form of meditation; some people clearly benefit while others less so. I harken back to the psychiatrist Dr. Schilder, who states in his book, "Hypnosis represents the pleasure of surrender."

At home, I continue to practice the relaxation techniques, and I listen to the CD in the evenings. Again I feel I am coming up short of my goal. I am not able to fully surrender. The office-based sessions and the guided CD hypnosis sessions lead to immediate relaxation. Unfortunately, the calm I derive from these sessions is short-lived. I continue to be plagued by restless sleep. I fall asleep fairly quickly, but I wake frequently throughout the night despite the hypnotist's suggestion to my subconscious that I would not be easily awakened, and if I did happen to wake up, I would fall quickly back to sleep. This has not been the case. With regard to my general level of anxiety and "Type A-ness," I perceive an increased level of calm immediately after the hypnosis sessions. Though, overall, I remain a stress monger. I have concluded that hypnosis for me is akin to meditation: when practiced, I achieve a state of deep relaxation. I had hoped to go even deeper and be able to have my subconscious manipulated, but I don't see this happening – not that I won't continue to try.

Enough about me. What proof is there that hypnosis works? Hypnotists claim they can cure smoking addiction, relieve pain, and strip one of all inhibitions. Where is the proof? Following is my attempt to summarize the medical literature on the benefits of hypnosis.

I return to my hypnotist's web page to begin my investigation. My hypnotist has solid academic credentials as a neuroscientist, and she has summarized several studies on hypnotherapy. Smoking appears to be a popular vice for which hypnotherapy is utilized. The website summarizes the results of six studies, all addressing smoking cessation via hypnosis. These studies found wild success in smoking cessation via hypnosis. Rates of abstinence from tobacco reach upwards of 90%. If true, these are impressive numbers. Traditional Western methods to stop smoking, such as nicotine patches, or medications such as Chantix, have only shown a 15-30% cessation rate. Any intervention with a success rate of 90% should be widely embraced; just imagine the lives that could be saved.

I do have one reservation when I review these studies: they are all in journals I have never heard of. Smoking cessation is a mainstream goal. I assume if a really convincing study had been performed and achieved a rate approaching 90%, it would be published in the *New England Journal of Medicine* or in a similarly prestigious journal, but these studies are published in the *International Journal of Clinical and Experimental Hypnosis* and in the *Journal of Nursing Scholarship.* I do a literature search of my own. I find several studies addressing hypnotherapy for smoking cessation. A Cochrane Database Review of the literature in 2010 finds "no evidence of a greater effect of hypnotherapy" when compared to other methods in achieving smoking cessation. In contrast, an article in the *American Journal of Medicine* in 2012 suggests hypnotherapy may help smokers quit, but no definitive conclusion could be made. I find these results sobering.

What about hypnosis for stress and anxiety? The benefits here are a bit harder to quantify. With smoking cessation, the results are black and white: either you quit smoking or you don't. In contrast, I doubt anyone can say they are ever completely free of anxiety. The studies reflect this nebulousness. Participants were classified as "significantly less anxious," and there was "compelling evidence" that hypnosis may help manage anxiety. Again, most of these studies were published in non-mainstream journals. The overall findings suggest benefit, but in my mind, remain inconclusive.

Pain management? Remember my hypnotist and her many tattoos? She confided to me that the experience of getting the tattoos was initially unbearably painful. When she got her first tattoo, she had to take repeated breaks due to the overwhelming pain. Subsequently, she used self-hypnosis while getting a tattoo and said the procedure became virtually pain free. Goodbye oxycodone, hello hypnosis. My research into this area again leaves me unsatisfied. Similar to studies of anxiety, studies of pain management rely on pain scales and subjective reports. I found several articles on using hypnosis to cope with labor pains during childbirth. Although several small studies show evidence of benefits for women receiving hypnosis regarding pain intensity, length of labor, and maternal hospital stay, the overall results are inconclusive. A large study, published in the Cochrane Database System Review, showed that women using self-hypnosis during childbirth required the same amount of epidural anesthesia to control labor pains as those who did not use hypnosis.

Hypnosis has been studied in many other realms. One interesting study evaluates post-hypnotic suggestion as a means to improve academic performance – it didn't. Another evaluates hypnosis to accelerate the healing of bone fractures – it did (although the study only had 12 subjects, 6 in the hypnotherapy group and 6 in the control group). There is a litany of other uses for hypnosis that range from treating headaches and menopausal symptoms, to curing obesity.

With all these potential benefits, why have I included hypnosis in my exploration of "alternative medicine?" Clearly, it should be mainstream. Perhaps psychiatry holds the answer.

My father-in-law, who is a very practical, educated mainstream psychiatrist, certainly believes hypnosis is real and can help treat his patients. I wonder about his colleagues. I come across an article published in 1962 in the *Journal of the American Medical Association*, the flagship journal for the AMA. Hypnosis was probably at its zenith in popularity around this time. In fact, only 46% of psychiatrists polled had experience with hypnosis, and a mere 13% used it in their practice. A more recent article published in 2010 by Dr. Robert London, a long-practicing psychiatrist, claims that hypnosis remains a "great therapeutic tool," and he laments its declining use by his profession. Dr. London also remarks that hypnosis does not work on everyone. He says, "If hypnotic strategies are going to work, they will be effective within a few sessions. If they do not work for a problem, it might be time to move on to other approaches."

Dr. London's words strike true. Despite my best efforts, I am struggling to see the benefits of hypnosis. It is time to move on.

## Hypnosis

**Cost of hypnosis session:** $50-$200

**Covered by standard insurance policies:** No, unless performed by a licensed psychiatrist.

**Published research:**

Smoking cessation: Studies with differing conclusions. A larger meta-analysis (review of prior published studies) found no benefit.[2] Yet a more recent meta-analysis in the *American Journal of Medicine* suggests benefit.[3]

Stress/Anxiety: Benefit shown in small randomized study.[4]

Pain management: Two studies evaluated hypnosis for labor pain. One found no benefit[5] while the second found possible benefit.[6]

Academic performance: No benefit.[7]

Healing of bone fractures: Maybe, but only evaluated in a very small pilot study of twelve patients.[8]

# Endnotes


1 Boyd R. Do People Only Use 10 Percent of Their Brains? *Scientific American.* Feb 7, 2008. http://www.scientificamerican.com/article/do-people-only-use-10-percent-of-their-brains/

2 Barnes, J., et al. Hypnotherapy for smoking cessation. *Cochrane Database Syst Rev*, 2010. 11:1-11.

3 Tahiri, M., et al. Alternative smoking cessation aids: a meta-analysis of randomized controlled trials. *Am J Med,*. 2012;125(6):576.

4 Cardena, E., et al. Hypnotic tape intervention ameliorates stress: a randomized, controlled study. *Int J Clin Exp Hypn*, 2013:61(2): 125-45.

5 Werner, A., et al. Self-hypnosis for coping with labor pain: a randomized controlled trial. *BJOG*, 2013 Feb:120(3):346-53.

6 Madden, K., et al. Hypnosis for pain management during labor and childbirth. *Cochrane Database Syst Rev,* 2012 Nov 14:11:CD009356.

7 Jacobson, N., et al. The effects of encoding in hypnosis and post-hypnotic suggestion on academic performance. *Am J Clin Hypn,* 2011 Apr;53(4):247-54.

8 Ginandes, C.S. & Rosenthal, D.I. Using hypnosis to accelerate the healing of bone fractures: a randomized controlled pilot study. *Altern Ther Health Med,* 1999 Mar;5(2):67-75.

# Chapter 15 The Cleanse (Not So Simple) – Detoxification Diets

Throughout my exploration of alternative therapies, I have intentionally avoided "detoxification diets," otherwise known as "cleanses." Why? I hate diets. Despite my aversion to any form of dietary restriction, I realize I am in the minority. A new cleanse or dietary fad seems to sprout every day, boasting every imaginable health benefit. I can no longer ignore the public's fascination with dietary cleansing. Therefore, in response to popular demand, I will subject myself, and my wife (if she is agreeable), to a cleanse.

What are the benefits of detoxification? Does my body need to be detoxified? To find the alternative medicine explanation, I once again turn to my guidebook, *Alternative Medicine – The Definitive Guide*. The authors state that "people . . . carry within their bodies a modern-day chemical cocktail derived from industrial chemicals, pesticides, food additives, heavy metals (like lead), . . . the residues of pharmaceuticals, legal drugs (alcohol, tobacco, caffeine), and illegal drugs." According to Dr. Haas, author of *The Detox Diet*, "Detoxification is instrumental for maintenance of the normal function and integrity of the intestinal flora and can enhance the natural ability of the body to resist infections, allergies, and skin disorders." I am surprised by the numerous purported health benefits of a cleanse. I always assumed weight loss was the primary goal.

With so many different types of cleanses advertised, how do I choose the one that is right for me? A quick Internet search reveals a litany of options. According to *iVillage*, among the "9 most popular cleanses" is "The Master Cleanse," which involves six to ten glasses per day of a mixture of maple syrup, lemon juice, water, cayenne pepper, lemonade, and a daily laxative. This is a favorite of both Demi Moore and Beyoncé. Other cleanses listed are the "Juju Cleanse," the "Candida Cleanse," the "Clean Program," and "Dr. Oz's 48-hour Cleanse." As I read the details of each cleanse, I find the majority of them to be either revolting or having the potential to starve me. A poll of my close friends adds a few other interesting options. My favorite is suggested by one of my close Cleveland buddies – the "Beer Diet." He claims it makes him "feel very slim and healthy, is a great boost to his confidence" (everything he says is funny or important), and it even makes him a better dancer at parties. Chris, my Aspen buddy, suggests eating only whole fruits and vegetables for seven days. He says if I combine this diet with rigorous exercise, I will go into ketosis (a metabolic process that occurs when the body does not have enough glucose for energy). Supposedly, that's good for you . . . if you survive.

After much consideration, I choose "The UltraSimple Diet," created by Dr. Mark Hyman. According to the cover of his book, it will: "Target your Belly Fat," "Revitalize your Health," and "Boost your Energy." My stepmother suggested this diet, and it does seem to meet all my criteria: It lasts only seven days (fourteen if you include the one week lead-in), it does not require commercial products (no "Dr. Hyman shakes" need be purchased), it does not include starvation, and daily enemas are not mandatory. It has just the right balance of kookiness and common sense that seems to typify the more popular diets. Better yet, my stepmother has given me a copy of the book. (One can also access the diet online.)

Don't worry, Dr. Hyman is not my colleague, and I am not getting any kickbacks for promoting his diet (at least not yet). My plan is to start off by completing his "Toxicity and Inflammation Quiz" so I can determine a before and after score. During the lead-in week, the goal is to cut out caffeine, processed and refined carbohydrates, high-fructose corn syrup, hydrogenated fats, processed foods, and alcohol. Even preparation for the diet sounds brutal. After the lead-in week, I will start the "UltraSimple Diet" in earnest. Let the suffering begin. When I emerge from this cleanse, I will be "detoxified" and hopefully revitalized. If this fails, I can always resort to the Beer Diet.

First, I fill out the "Toxicity and Inflammation Quiz." My score is 16. This gives me a health status of "mild imbalance." This seems about right. Now if it were a mental health score, I am not so sure. According to Dr. Hyman, persons with a mild health imbalance might expect the UltraSimple Diet to lead to "improved digestion, better skin, and less nasal congestion." Fortunately, I don't suffer from any of these maladies at the moment. As my friends can attest, I could have used "better skin" when I was in high school. Then my facial acne was so severe, my face looked like it had been "attacked by a swarm of bees" – to quote my brother. Hopefully, I will at least see "increased energy and improved mood." Weight loss is also a possible benefit, which I don't need, having inherited the "skinny" gene from my mother. The areas where I score poorly are 1) "belching and passing gas" (although I don't see this as a problem, my wife has a different opinion – perhaps I have submitted her to one too many "fart tents" at night); 2) "headaches," which still occur with regularity, but are rarely disabling; and 3) "insomnia," which I have described in prior chapters. In addition to the quiz, I record my starting weight of 192 lbs.

In accordance with Dr. Hyman's instructions, on Sunday my wife and I embark on the one-week "preparation" leading up to the UltraSimple Diet. It is difficult to resist drinking a beer while watching Sunday Night Football, but I do. Our plan is to systematically cut out all toxin-laden foods over the course of the week. I decide to stop alcohol and caffeine cold turkey. On Monday, I pay for my decision. I substitute a glass of orange juice for coffee in the morning, and at 11 a.m., I have a crushing headache. Work is a chore. I eye the Coke on my colleague's desk and consider wrestling it away from him, but somehow I persevere. The rest of the day is a headachy blur. I tuck myself in at 9:30 p.m. and hope that Tuesday will be a better day. As I reflect back on the day, I am not sure that the lack of caffeine is totally to blame. I am also missing my normal boluses of sugar-laden food: no Luna bar at mid-morning, no cookies with lunch, no cookies when I get home, and no cookies at night. You get the picture. Tuesday promises to be a better day. I decide to substitute green tea for my usual coffee – at least this has some caffeine in it. Not too tasty, but again, at this point, who cares about taste? I can feel a headache threatening to break through, but at 2 p.m. on Tuesday, it has yet to take over.

During the rest of the week, I successfully eliminate caffeine and processed sugars from my diet. By mid-week, I jettison the green tea. Although it has a bit of caffeine (equivalent to a half cup of java), it is not worth suffering its bland taste and the nausea it induces. I am not perfect. God forbid, I eat a turkey sandwich on wheat bread for lunch one day, even though this is a double violation – processed meat and a wheat product. By and large, though, I am faithful to Dr. Hyman's instructions. I certainly would enjoy a beer or two after some particularly trying days at work, but I abstain. Not that I am trying, but I have already lost a few pounds. A week has passed, the lead-in is over, and now the heavy lifting begins: the cleanse.

As I begin the cleanse, I must give thanks – or perhaps blame is more appropriate – to my wife. She makes this cleanse possible. Not only is she detoxing with me, but she has done the majority of shopping and food preparation for the coming week. Looking over our bill from Whole Foods reminds me that "health food" is not cheap, at least not at this time of year. Earlier in the summer, we likely could have purchased most of the veggies at a farmers' market, but as we move into fall, the selection of inexpensive produce has evaporated. The bill for a bunch of veggies (that I typically abhor), rice protein powder, and flax seed is over $100. Even more appalling to my penny-pinching sensibilities is that these expensive, unfamiliar vegetables (radish root, winter squash, kale, chard, seaweed) are the key ingredients of the UltraBroth, which is a staple of the UltraSimple Diet. Preparation of the UltraBroth entails cooking these veggies in a large pot of boiling water for sixty minutes and then discarding them and only keeping the broth. My goodness! I am not sure if I am more shocked by the waste or relieved that I don't have to eat the veggies. The end result is a pot of yellow-gray "broth" which resembles dishwater both in appearance and taste. I can hardly wait for my 2-4 cups a day.

Although the UltraSimple diet has barely begun, I can already tell it will not be so simple. Fortunately, one area I don't have to worry about is having regular bowel movements. Dr. Hyman devotes several pages of his book to the merits of frequent stools and the horrors of constipation. In fact, according to the UltraSimple diet, if you have failed to have a bowel movement by 10 a.m., you are supposed to take an herbal laxative. I chuckle when I bring this to my wife's attention. It is already 11 in the morning, and she has failed to go. I see a laxative in someone's near future. On the other hand, I have absolutely no worries about meeting the 10 a.m. cut-off. Ever since my time in Ghana, West Africa, I have multiple loose stools every morning. I tease my boys by claiming I am infested with intestinal worms that I picked up in Africa. For all I know, it may be true.

Breakfast consists of some lemon juice in hot water followed by an UltraShake. The shake is basically a water-based fruit smoothie. It contains a blend of non-citrus fruit, rice protein powder, flaxseed, and water. The flaxseed gives it a not so palatable odor, but it is drinkable. I tolerate the shake, but I yearn for my normal weekend breakfast of coffee, eggs, toast, and orange juice with bacon on the side. Around 10 a.m., I am ready for my standard mid-morning snack. Instead of my usual energy bar, I have a cup of UltraBroth – ouch. After a lunch of bland sautéed veggies over brown rice and some leftover UltraShake, I am downright cranky. This week is going to last forever. My nightmares will be full of UltraShakes and UltraBroths. Fortunately, there is one part of the UltraSimple Diet that is not so bad . . . the UltraBath. A long soak in a hot bath with Epsom salts, baking soda, and lavender oil is something to look forward to. I might just drink the bath water when I am done, or would that be UltraDisgusting?

The week passes in a monotonous blur. I scale back on exercise to conserve energy. I fear that if I bike to work, I may not have the strength to bike up the mountain on the way home. Each day, I consume more UltraShakes and UltraBroth. The diet allows unlimited UltraBroth, but it is little consolation. I find myself daydreaming about food – hot buttered rolls, a cup of coffee, a thick, juicy steak, or even a candy bar. I sorely miss my standard fare of a meat and cheese sandwich and some peanut butter crackers at lunch. Instead, I eat rice with sautéed veggies – not an adequate substitute in my mind. Undoubtedly, the rice and veggies are healthier, but it leaves my stomach aching for more. My friends give me encouragement, but I can only weakly acknowledge their support. I mistakenly expected to reach a state of nirvana. My detoxified body is supposed to be brimming with energy like a filly ready to romp in a dew-covered field in the morning. Instead, I feel like an old man starving on a deserted island.

It is Sunday once again. The UltraSimple Diet is over and not a minute too soon. I am losing weight at a frightening pace. Skinny when I started this endeavor, I am now downright emaciated. I lost a total of twelve pounds – four pounds during the week lead-in phase, and eight more while following the UltraSimple Diet. The last time I was this thin, I had just returned from eight months in West Africa (and no, I did not contract Ebola). Getting dressed in the morning is a challenge. What clothes do I have that won't swallow me up and make me look like a bag of bones?

Dr. Hyman claims that by "reducing toxic stress" through his UltraSimple diet, I will feel renewed and rejuvenated. Is it true? Maybe. The past two weeks of no processed sugar, no wheat products, no caffeine, and no alcohol has certainly changed my attitude toward food. I realize now that most of my diet in the past has been made up of synthesized, unnatural foods. Despite the change in my perspective, I do plan on eating many of these foods again, but in moderation. Additionally, I will be adding many more fruits and veggies to my diet. If the UltraSimple Diet is meant to reboot one's attitude towards food and inspire healthy eating, then it scored a ten.

Do I feel less toxic? Not really. What I felt for the past two weeks is a deep, rumbling hunger. Let's get this straight, being hungry is not fun. I no longer aspire to be on a reality survival show. I want to know where and when my next meal will be. In addition to my newfound respect for food, I learned to tolerate pangs of hunger and will no longer require a fistful of cookies to stave it off. Although I now appreciate the merits of sautéed veggies on brown rice, I don't think I need to eat this particular combination again for a few months. I also don't see any more UltraBroths in my future. This morning, I happily sat down to a breakfast of scrambled eggs, toast, and turkey bacon. Give me some credit – I had hot water with lemon rather than my usual cup of coffee.

I retake the "Toxicity and Inflammation" quiz outlined in the UltraSimple Diet manual. My pre-diet score was a 16, which rated me as having a "mild imbalance." My post-diet score is little changed at 13. Where did my score improve? For the past week, I have not had any heartburn, belching, or passage of gas. Amazing. I can't say I really care whether I pass gas or not, but my wife is thankful to be spared. The one area where my score worsened was general fatigue. For some reason, the feeling of starvation also made me feel more sluggish and averse to exercise. Imagine that.

What is my assessment of the whole detoxification process? The diet is a bit over the top. I don't plan on doing a cleanse like this one again. If rapid weight loss is your goal, then the UltraSimple Diet is great. My wife lost six pounds, and my colleague at work lost five pounds and a few clothing sizes. I lost over twelve pounds. I imagine I passed beyond the stage of breaking down fat to digesting my own muscles. Perhaps I even developed ketosis – my friend Chris will be proud. I will now go about trying to regain some of the weight I lost. As for the benefit of this diet and ones like it for reducing toxicity and inflammation, I remain skeptical. I feel as inflamed today as I felt two weeks ago, and this is despite the fact I largely abstained from vigorous exercise. It is hard to go for a long bike ride or lift weights when you are craving food. Despite my sufferings, I am glad I joined the multitude of cleansing veterans. My liver must be smiling. While I may not have become a cleansing devotee, I do admit it has effectively reset my attitude toward food.

## Detoxification (Cleanse)

**Cost of a cleanse:** Most are available online for free or passed around by word of mouth. (The true cost is more physical than economic.)

**Covered by standard insurance policies:** No

**Published research:** (not much)

Published findings: A handful of small and methodologically flawed studies suggests that detox diets enhance liver detoxification and eliminate organic pollutants from the body. There are no randomized controlled studies assessing the effectiveness of detox diets in humans.[1]

# Endnote

1 Klein, A.V. & Kiat. H. Review: Detox diets for toxin elimination and weight management: a critical review of the evidence. *J Hum Nutr Diet*, 2014:1-12.

# Chapter 16 Don't Touch My Dosha – Ayurvedic Medicine

For my next foray into alternative medicine, I will travel back in time and give Ayurvedic medicine a try. Ayurveda is one of the world's oldest forms of holistic healing. Ayurveda traces its origins back thousands of years to ancient India. The first question that comes to mind as I learn about this new discipline is how do you pronounce Ayurvedic? Is it Aar-oovadick? Ayorveedak? Fortunately, I don't have to look far to find clarification. I share my office with Dr. Gupta, not the world-famous Sanjay Gupta, but Vinnie Gupta. Dr. Gupta informs me the correct pronunciation is "Eye yur VAY dick." Now that I can pronounce Ayurvedic, I am ready to find a local practitioner. Now that I live in Asheville, North Carolina, home of all things alternative, I am sure I will have several options to choose from. San Francisco has nothing on my little mountain town when it comes to non-traditional forms of medicine. Had I searched for an Ayurvedic doctor in Cleveland, Ohio, the city where I started this quest, I would have been out of luck. Asheville, on the other hand, not only has Ayurveda, but it boasts one of the few Ayurvedic centers in the United States. Don't lose heart, Clevelanders – a Case Western-University Hospitals affiliate in Cleveland is adding Ayurveda as a wellness option, further proof that alternative medicine is not really so "alternative" any longer.

What is Ayurveda? Does a form of wellness therapy invented thousands of years ago still have relevance in modern times? To answer these questions, I turn to my usual sources: *Alternative Medicine – The Definitive Guide,* and WebMD. These two sources provide viewpoints from opposite sides of the spectrum – alternative medicine devotees versus Western-trained doctors like me. According to Dr. Deepak Chopra, Ayurvedic physicians ask, "Who is my patient?" rather than "What disease does my patient have?" The focus of Ayurveda is to promote good health rather than to treat disease. Ayurveda believes in the connectedness of everything in the universe (*connectedness* is a key buzzword for many "alternative" beliefs). Ayurveda says everything is composed of the five basic elements: space, air, water, fire, and earth (a bit simpler than the 118 elements that make up the Periodic Table).* These basic elements combine to form a person's metabolic type, or *dosha*. One's dosha is quite important because if your dosha is out of balance, you are prone to illness.

I research the three doshas: Vata, Pitta, and Kapha. Which one am I? Persons typically are of one predominant dosha, but may express the other doshas to a lesser degree (this reminds me a bit of astrology). There are certain characteristics associated with each dosha. My "bible," *Alternative Medicine*, lists traits associated with each dosha. As I read the general traits associated with each dosha, I am reminded of horoscopes, which give general predictions that could apply to everyone. Despite my initial cynicism, I am clearly a Pitta: medium build; fair-thin hair (thinner than I would like); warm-perspiring skin; doesn't miss a meal; lives by the clock; intelligent and articulate (of course); orderly-efficient; warm and loving (maybe); short-tempered (nope); heartburn (yep); hemorrhoids (yes, how embarrassing); and acne (my friends definitely remember my pizza-faced youth). Wow – after reading the list, I have no doubt that I am a Pitta through and through.

---

* This concept of five basic elements dates back to the pre-scientific concept in Ancient Greece, which proposed that ether, air, water, fire, and earth were the building blocks of all matter.[1] Science has proven that the ancient systems were incorrect. The atomic theory is the correct explanation, which classifies atoms into the elements of the Periodic Table.

According to WebMD, those with Pitta as their primary life force are more likely to develop anger and negative emotions (bullshit! I hate this website!), Crohn's disease (I do have bowel issues), heart disease, heartburn, high blood pressure, and infections. Fortunately, I am an infectious diseases doctor, so I should be able to handle the last of these. Based on my overwhelming Pitta-ness, I should have had a least one cardiac bypass surgery by now. I don't dare wait any longer. I need to find guidance before I croak. I will set up my first Ayurvedic consultation right away.

A week passes before I manage to carve out a couple of hours to see the Ayurvedic doctor for an initial consultation. Ayurveda is pure Asheville – funky, earthy, and alternative. I expect the Ayurveda center to be located downtown in a trendy area, but no, I am shocked to find it is located in a modern office space on Hendersonville Road. Imagine big box stores, Bennigan's, excessive signage, and traffic congestion, and you have Hendersonville Road – the least appealing area of Asheville. Surprisingly, the Ayurvedic center is not the only alternative option in this area. The very same office building also houses an integrative medicine clinic – just one more sign that alternative medicine has gone mainstream.

I expect this visit might be expensive. I harken back to my visit to the Naturopath: The initial consultation cost over $100, yet this was only a small expense relative to the cost of the recommended herbs and homeopathic remedies. Blue Cross and Blue Shield is not taken here. I know that herbal remedies are a big part of Ayurveda. I can only imagine the price tag. Herbs purchased in a grocery store are expensive enough, but import them from India and prescribe them as a remedy, and I am sure the cost skyrockets.

I enter the Ayurveda center, and no one is there to greet me. I can tell by the Indian pictures on the wall, the dim lights, and the wicker furniture that I am in the right place. A sign on a table says someone will be out shortly. I take a seat and try to channel my inner Buddha. Look at me – Mister Low-Key, not in a hurry. In truth, I am analyzing everything. I can only aspire to be Type B. Fifteen minutes after my consultation is scheduled to begin, a customer emerges from the back room, followed by Jesus. Not actually Jesus, but certainly a reasonable modern-day imitation. The doctor (previously referred to as Jesus) has long hair pulled back into a ponytail, a loose-fitting shirt, jeans, and no shoes. He is clearly in his element. He is a true Ashevillean, while I am just an imposter. He invites me to the back room. We sit across from one another in two upright chairs. His office combines modernity with ancient India. There is a table top with a computer, books, and his scribblings juxtaposed with pictures of India; a waist-high, golden elephant Buddha; and shelves stocked with large jars of crushed herbs. This is a far cry from the sterile hospital dispensary with which I am familiar.

After casually introducing himself, the doctor launches into the usual questions that begin any visit: "What brings you here?" "What do you hope to gain?" He then begins a fairly detailed inquisition into my dietary habits, lifestyle, and my general constitution. I expected this line of questioning. Of course, what he really wants to discover is my dosha. Should I save him the effort and just blurt out that "I am a Pitta." I suppress the urge and answer his questions faithfully. "Yes, I sweat a lot. No, I am not prone to constipation. In fact, I have frequent loose stools. Yes, I would describe myself as high stress. I suffer from insomnia, heartburn, and headaches." These last two admissions pique his interest. He does not seem surprised that I get heartburn. He delves deeper into my headaches – "How frequent are they? What triggers them? How do you relieve them?"

Next he takes a very detailed history of my dietary habits. I tell him about the cleanse that I just recently completed, and he nods approvingly. In fact, I think the cleanse has stolen much of his thunder. He recommends avoiding empty sweets – done; caffeine – done; processed foods – done. I am becoming worried. It appears that if I follow his dietary recommendations, the cleanse, which I am relieved is over, will live on minus the dreaded UltraBroth. Fortunately, he doesn't mention cutting out alcohol. I am not sure if this is an oversight, but I don't ask. I can drink my evening glass of wine or beer. Hallelujah!

Now that history taking is completed, we come to the physical examination. Where will he probe? What bodily samples will I have to produce? He pulls up his chair until we are directly across from one another, and our knees are nearly touching. He places a square pillow as a bridge across our laps. First, he stares deeply into my eyes. Then he has me stick out my tongue while he studies its furrows and ridges. I wonder if the cleft I have from biting through my tongue as an infant gives him any insight. Then he has me place my arms on the pillows, and he uses three fingers to check the pulses on both my wrists. Apparently, he is much more adept at reading one's pulse than I am. I remember reading about Ayurvedic doctors being able to appreciate three components of one's pulse and thereby deriving inferences regarding overall well-being. After a few more seconds of pulse reading, he is done. The exam is done. No urine or blood sample required.

He declares my constitution is Pitta. I am amazed. He also says my "imbalanced state" is also Pitta, but with a bit of Vata. Now that my dosha is revealed, he can tailor a specific therapeutic plan for me.

He returns his focus to my diet. We spend extensive time going over foods I should avoid and foods I should load up on.

He encourages me to double my water intake to two liters a day. (It seems that every discipline, including Western medicine, is convinced that we are continually at risk of dehydration.) I am to avoid drinking milk in close proximity to when I drink orange juice. Most of his dietary recommendations are fairly standard: Avoid processed foods and increase my intake of natural fruits and veggies.

He says that Pittas have a lot of heat; therefore, I need to avoid heat-producing foods, which will feed my fire. He is pleased by my frequent bowel movements, but remains concerned about my headaches and heartburn. He says heartburn is a symptom rather than a disease itself. When I express an openness to try herbal remedies, he smiles. He leaps up, stares at his shelves, and contemplates out loud which jars hold the right herbs for me. He grabs a Ziploc baggie and starts adding a scoop or two of various herbal powders. After a few moments of indecision, followed by a few clarifying questions regarding my sleep habits and bowel movements, he completes the herbal concoction and hands me the bag. He tells me to take two teaspoons twice daily mixed with hot water.

The visit is coming to an end. He suggests I contact him via email in a week or two to report on my progress and possibly to schedule a visit to the Ayruvedic day spa for an Abhyanga (warm oil massage) or perhaps a Shirodhara (Ayurvedic Bliss Therapy). He says these treatments are part of the process to restore balance and promote relaxation. The next question – cash or credit card? Alas, my bliss is coming to an end. The total bill is $150 for the consultation and a mere $20 for the herbs. Compared to my naturopathic visit, I am making out like a bandit.

Once I get home, I am ready to address my dosha imbalance. The Ayurvedic doctor told me both my Pitta and Vata doshas are out of whack. With such an imbalance, one might expect I would have a hard time functioning, but somehow I have managed. After eating a regular diet for the past week while recovering from my UltraSimple cleanse, I am ready to follow the Ayurvedic recommendations. According to WebMD, "[a] main goal of Ayurvedic medicine is to cleanse your body of undigested food . . . which can stick inside your body and make you sick." Now I understand why the doctor was so pleased by my regular bowel movements: I don't think anything sticks to my intestines. Nevertheless, I am embarking on a panchakarma, or cleansing process. Hopefully, this will correct my imbalance and create harmony among my doshas.

There are many methods to a successful panchakarma. Methods include bleeding, massage, cathartics, and enemas. I vote no to the bleeding. Fortunately, I didn't see any leeches in the doctor's office. A good massage, however, I might be willing to endure. Other treatments may include aromatherapy, dietary modifications, herbs, lifestyle changes, yoga, and meditation. My doctor has chosen diet and herbs for the first go around. This will be followed by an Ayurvedic Rasayana Day Spa package to complete my panchakarma.

Following the doctor's advice, I once again eliminate caffeine from my diet. He suggested green tea as an alternative, but I now associate green tea with my recently completed UltraSimple Diet and even the thought of it brings on a wave of nausea. Besides, I will be drinking hot water with a teaspoon of crushed Ayurvedic herbs mixed in twice a day. Surely this will be better than green tea. In addition to the crushed herbal concoction, I once again cut out the "empty sweets" which I so adore – not an easy feat in the wake of Halloween. I am loading up on veggies, nuts, and fruits – boy, this feels familiar. I can certainly appreciate the logic behind this diet. It is basically a healthier version of my regular diet. I do cheat a bit, but on the balance, I am eating pretty healthy. I have no complaints, except for those herbs. Do the powdered herbs mixed in a cup of hot water really taste better than green tea? No, they do not. The crushed herbs take the form of a gray powder. The powder reminds me of ashes from someone's cremation – perhaps this is where crematoriums sell their unclaimed bodies. I mix one teaspoon of the herbal concoction in a cup of steaming water. With vigorous stirring, I can almost get the herbs to dissolve. On its own, it is undrinkable; once I add freshly squeezed lemon, it is just bearable. The result is a gray, slightly noxious, gritty drink. I manage to force it down twice a day.

If the appearance and taste of this gritty herbal drink is not enough to discourage me from taking the herbs, then perhaps an article published in the *Journal of the American Medical Society* (JAMA) in 2007 should have done the trick. The authors found that several Indian manufactured Ayurvedic products might result in lead and/or mercury ingestions 100-10,000 times acceptable limits. In case you are unfamiliar with lead and mercury, they are heavy metals that can cause life-threatening illnesses when ingested. The Federal Drug Administration has warned that 20% of Ayurvedic medicines contain toxic metals, including lead, mercury, and arsenic. Yes, that is right, arsenic* – the poison beautiful young wives use to murder their old rich husbands.

Despite the above warnings, I stick to the diet and take my herbal remedy. My son Connor is very worried about the potential heavy metal poisoning that seems to be looming. He has reviewed the symptoms of lead poisoning (abdominal pain, constipation, headache, confusion, irritability), mercury poisoning (tremors, inflamed gums, increased salivation, psychiatric symptoms), and arsenic poisoning (nausea, vomiting,

---

* Arsenic and mercury were used (and recommended) in Western medicine in the 19th century. The arsenic gave patients a flushed sensation, a feeling that something was really happening (only it wasn't good).

diarrhea, hair loss, rash). He is monitoring me closely. Other than going bald and acting a bit crazy, I haven't changed a bit. Connor is struggling with determining which symptoms he should attribute to the herbs and which ones are typical for his father.

One week into the diet, I feel pretty good. The herbs do scare me a bit, but I am betting the herbs I got fall in the 80% that are free of heavy metals. I feel healthier by the day. I am sure that my doshas are smiling.

After completing a second week of dieting and Ayurvedic herbs, I am ready for some hands-on therapy. I arrange a Rasayana Day Spa appointment. Finding an open appointment time is the hardest part. Apparently, Ayurvedic medicine, like other forms of alternative medicine, is quite popular in Asheville. The first appointment I can arrange is two weeks away. Finally, the day arrives. Much to my delight, the Ayurvedic center has relocated to the North side of Asheville. As I pull up in my car, I appreciatively note that the center is now in a turn-of-the-century home in an eclectic area of town. I like it when my preconceived notions are realized. This is much better than the commercial section of town where it previously sat. I arrive at 12:30 p.m. on the dot. Despite my aspiration to be more laid back, I hope I am not forced to wait – I am playing hooky from work, and I don't want to be gone too long. I toss my pager in the front console of my car and beseech it to remain silent for the next two hours. I also turn off my phone. Receiving pages and calls from the hospital will not help me relax.

Again, the reception area is empty. I sink into a comfortable couch in the front room. The smell of incense wafts through the building. A sign alerts me that a session is in progress. After only a few minutes, the Ayurvedic doctor beckons me to follow him upstairs. The Ayurvedic office is located in the front room of the house on the second floor. There is a massage table in the center of the room and Indian art on the walls. I see the shelves of crushed herbs made the trip, as well as the three-foot high elephant Buddha. The doctor asks how I feel and if I have been following the dietary prescription he suggested. I say that I have. I mention that the herbs are not so tasty. He says their smell and texture are part of the therapy. He is not opposed to my adding lemon juice to the mixture of hot water and herbs, as I have been doing, but says I should also experience the herbs on their own (no way in hell, I think to myself). He then introduces me to his female assistant, and we get down to business. They step out of the room while I fully undress and cover myself with a warm cover while lying on the massage table.

Upon their return, gentle music is turned on – piano, followed by various reed instruments – quite soothing. Over the next hour, I experience the abhyanga (warm herbal oil massage). The two practitioners work in unison – one starting on my head and face and the other on my feet. I am squeamish about anyone touching the bottoms of my feet. Usually, the experience is anything but relaxing. Amazingly, I tolerate it and even like it. Perhaps having one person kneading my scalp while the soles of my feet are massaged provides the necessary tactile distraction. He even massages my ears. He places mint drops (or something similar) in my nose to open my sinuses. The next hour is decadent: two sets of hands rubbing me from stem to stern, front and back with warm herbal oil. I have never received such attention. I later read the oil is a liquid form of fat that is well absorbed through the skin. Purportedly, it enters one's circulation and binds to toxins, which are eliminated through normal processes. This form of detoxification sure beats the heck out of the Ultra-Simple Diet I did last month. The hour rapidly passes. When it is over, I reluctantly move on to the next stage of my day spa package, the bashpa swedana, or herbal steam bath.

The doctor leads me, still fully disrobed except for what appears to be a small hand towel, to a single-person sauna in the corner of the room. The front of the steam bath swings open to reveal a small bench. The door is closed, and my whole body is enveloped, except for my head. Slowly, steam emanates from the floor of the chamber. It is nice and warm. I wish I had one of these at home. It is a bit strange though: while my body is bathed in steam, my head is out in the room just hanging out. It reminds me of the Halloween gag of the talking head poking through a table as if it is the main course for dinner. Meanwhile, the Ayurvedic doctor and his helper are milling around the room setting up for the next stage of my experience. It gives me a chance to ask some questions. I ask, "Where do you get the jars of powdered herbs?" and "Have you traveled to India?" He replies some of the herbs are purchased from U.S.- based companies, while he acquires others through his sources in India. (My fears are realized . . . Indian herbs . . . toxic metals – I try not to show my concern.) He has spent time in India, and his mentors are native Indians who trained him here in the United States.

I then ask about the other Ayurvedic methods of cleansing I read about – bleeding, emetics, and laxatives. He says he uses all of these methods, but only for special cases. He explains that in India, leeches are often used, but here in the U.S., he just encourages patients to donate blood and to adhere to a diet of cleansing herbs.

He says that dermatologic conditions respond particularly well to bleeding* while emetics, or herbs that induce vomiting, are useful for treating conditions such as gastric reflux disease. He also uses laxatives. The goal of all of these therapies is to help remove toxins, or alma, from

---

* Bloodletting dates back to Ancient Greece when it was believed to be a method for draining one of evil humors. It was subsequently discredited, and finally vanished from modern medicine with the discovery of antibiotics.[2]

one's system. He says that with most of his clients he primarily focuses on dietary changes, herbal meds, and day spa treatments, such as I have been receiving. Deprived of leeches and emetics, it appears I have been receiving "Panchakarma– lite." This is fine with me, but it is fascinating to learn that the more "alternative" aspects of Ayurvedic medicine are fully embraced even here in Asheville. After about 20 minutes in the steam bath, I am ready for my final treatment of the day, a shirodhara.

Shirodhara involves slowly pouring liquid over one's head (shiro). *Dhara* means "flow." I return to the massage table, and the assistant dims the lights and places a small, wet towel over my eyes. The soothing music is resumed, and over the next 30 minutes, warm sesame seed oil is slowly poured over my forehead. The oil is released from a suspended pot that resembles a honeypot with a nozzle on the bottom. The oil runs over my forehead and then oozes through my hair and is collected in a basin below my head and recycled. The doctor says most people find it very relaxing and are able to enter a meditative state. He is not kidding. Here I am, lying naked on a table with only a thin sheet covering me while a stranger pours oil over my head, and I actually fall asleep – unprecedented. Eventually, the music stops, and I wake up. I sit on the edge of the table for a few minutes to get my bearings, and then I wrap myself in the sheet and walk to a shower. Once in the bathroom I look in the mirror, and the reflection shows a person who appears ready to audition for the movie *Grease*.

After a quick shower, I pay my bill, a cool $199, but well worth it, and I drive back to work. I have completed my Rasayana Day Spa. I am very relaxed, borderline comatose, in fact. Fortunately, the rest of the afternoon is not too taxing. I don't think I could have handled any difficult tasks this afternoon.

After one more week of diet and herbs, my month-long flirtation with Ayurvedic medicine has come to an end. During the past month I have completed a pared-down version of a panchakarma, or cleansing. I consider the approach that I have taken to be a Western adaptation of the real thing. With the guidance of the Ayurvedic doctor, I focused on dietary changes, herbal supplements, and a day spa treatment. The more adventurous panchakarmas might include purgatives, enemas, and bleeding by leeches. While the path I took may have lacked the excitement of a good bleeding, it still had its moments. The shirodhara, which involved the slow, sustained pouring of warm oil over my forehead, was soothing and unlike any of my prior experiences. I feared my enjoyment of shirodhara would be offset by a raging crop of acne pustules in my scalp the following week, but fortunately, I was spared this embarrassment.

Is Ayurveda worth the time and money? Yes and no. Perhaps if my dosha (life-force) had been more out of balance, I would have been more aware of the results. Aside from the utter relaxation I experienced during my day spa experience, I am unable to appreciate any objective changes in my overall well-being. I appear to have survived the daily herbal ingestions despite the real possibility of heavy metal poisoning. I will not miss my twice daily doses of the powdered herbs, which look and taste like cremation remains – dearly departed "old aunt Louise," I like to joke. The dietary recommendations, which include increasing intake of fruit and veggies, avoiding processed foods, and limiting caffeine, all make sense for one's overall health.

While my personal anecdotes are fine, you may be wondering if there is any proof that Ayurveda is beneficial. To answer this question, I hit the books (really, the computer because who really uses books for research any longer?). First, I investigate the claims that the herbal oil massage can enter the circulation and bind toxins – I come up empty. That is not to say that Ayurvedic might not have benefits. There is evidence certain Ayurvedic herbs can effectively lower both short- and long-term blood sugars in diabetics. The use of Diabecon, one of the commonly prescribed Ayurvedic herbs, not only lowers blood sugars, but leads to increases in circulating insulin. Another study compared Ayurvedic medicine to methotrexate, a commonly accepted therapy of Western medicine for the treatment of rheumatoid arthritis. This was a small study, only 43 patients, but it was double-blinded and placebo-controlled (two critical components for a well-done clinical study), and it showed the two therapies had equivalent benefit.[3] In other work, varieties of the herb boswellia, otherwise known as frankincense, were found to produce a resin with anti-inflammatory effects in the lab. Preliminary clinical trial results suggest boswellia may benefit those with osteoarthritis (classic old-age arthritis). Despite these positive findings, the majority of research is inconclusive, and definitive proof that Ayurveda is beneficial has remained elusive. Proponents of Ayurveda will point out that a main tenet of Ayurveda is the focus on the individual, leading to highly tailored regimens based on one's particular needs. Thus, the gold standard of double-blinded, placebo-controlled experimentation runs contrary to Ayurvedic principles and might not give accurate results. Although this argument has some merit, I find for a discipline practiced by a majority of the Indian population for thousands of years, the proof is not convincing.

While there is a paucity of data supporting benefit, the potential risk in taking Ayurvedic medicines derived from Indian sources is very real. An analysis of Ayurvedic medicines published in the *Journal of the American Medical Association* in 2008 found 21% of Ayurvedic medications contained dangerous levels of lead, mercury, and/or arsenic.[4] A 2012 report from the Center for Disease Control described six cases of lead poisoning in pregnant women in New York City due to ingestion of Ayurvedic medications originating in India.[5] They found lead concentrations as high as 2.4% of the total medication as well as mercury and arsenic. Needless to say, lead exposure is bad for both mother and baby. Fetal lead exposure increases the risk for low birth weight, reduced intelligence, and behavioral problems.

To sum it up: Ayurveda definitely promotes many beneficial habits – improved diet, massage, yoga, and relaxation – but, keep an eye on those herbs. I will try to continue the diet and perhaps repeat the day spa, but I will leave the herbal ashes for the diehards (no pun intended).

## Ayurveda

**Cost of consultation:** $50-$250 (depending on length of visit)

**Cost of Ayurvedic Spa Packages**: $50-$100 for single treatment, $200-$500 for ½ to full day of treatments, $3,000-4,600 for week-long Panchakarma programs

**Cost of herbs**: $20-$50

**Covered by standard insurance policies:** No

**Published research:**

Osteoarthritis: A review of 19 randomized and 14 non-randomized controlled studies found support for the use of the herbs Rumalaya and Shunti-Guduchi for treatment of osteoarthritis, but other herbs studied had negative results or were inconclusive.[6]

Rheumatoid Arthritis: A small, single, randomized controlled study showed equal efficacy of Ayurveda as compared to methotrexate.[3]

Diabetes: A published review found significant glucose-lowering effects of some herbal mixtures, but due to small sample sizes and methodologic deficiencies, no conclusions could be drawn regarding their efficacy.[7]

According to the National Center for Complementary and Alternative Medicine, there are not enough well-controlled clinical trials and systematic research reviews to prove Ayurvedic approaches are beneficial. [8]

Risks: An article published in *JAMA* found several Indian-manufactured Ayurvedic products could result in heavy metal ingestions 100 to 10,000 times greater than acceptable limits.[4]

# Endnotes


1 Boyd, T.J.M. & Sanderson, J.J. (2003). *The physics of plasmas*. Cambridge University Press, p. 1.

2 Thomas, D.P. The demise of bloodletting. *J R Coll Physicians Edinb,* 2014; 44:72–7.

3 Furst, D.E., et al. Double-blind, randomized, controlled, pilot study comparing classic Ayurvedic medicine, methotrexate, and their combination in rheumatoid arthritis. *J Clin Rehumatol,* 2011 June: 17(4):185-92.

4 Saper, R.B., et al. Lead, mercury, and arsenic in US- and Indian-manufactured Ayurvedic medicines sold via the Internet. *JAMA,* 2008;300(8):915-923.

5 CDC. Lead poisoning in pregnant women who used Ayurvedic medications from India — New York City, 2011–2012. *MMWR,* 2012; 61(33);641-646.

6 Kessler, C.S., et al. Ayurvedic interventions for osteoarthritis: a systematic review and meta-analysis. *Rheumat Int,* 2015 Feb:35 (2):211-32.

7 Sridharan, K., et al. Ayurvedic treatments for diabetes mellitus. *Cochrane Database of Systemic Reviews,* 2011:12

8 National Center for Complementary and Alternative Medicine (NCAM) website: "Ayurvedic medicine: an introduction."

# Chapter 17 The Power of Rocks – Crystal Therapy

My self-described "bible," *Alternative Medicine – The Definitive Guide*, has failed me for the first time. Nowhere within its over one thousand pages can I find a reference to "healing with crystals." Surely I can learn more about the subject on the National Center for Alternative and Complementary Medicine's website, but no, I strike out once again. Maybe I have finally found a truly "alternative" alternative. Fortunately, once again Asheville does not let me down. There is an abundance of sites within town that offer healing with crystals. What is crystal healing? According to reputable sources, crystal healing is a technique using crystals and other stones as conduits for natural healing energy. Each crystal has unique properties that can benefit certain conditions or illnesses. A common belief is that crystals stimulate our body's "chakras," seven points of energy along our bodies that start on the forehead and extend down to the pelvis. Each chakra's name is based on the corresponding region of the body – sacral chakra, solar plexus chakra, heart chakra, and so forth. Certain crystals work with certain chakras.

I perform an exhaustive Internet search for "crystals," "crystal healing," and "crystal therapy" in the Asheville region and devise a plan. I have created my own pu pu platter of crystal samplings. I will begin my journey with a visit to Michele, who offers the world-renowned "John of God Crystal Bed Therapy." The crystal bed promises deep relaxation and increased energy along with a "redefined sense of life purpose." I will follow this up with an excursion to the Asheville Salt Cave. The cave contains 20 tons of "crystal salt" with all 84 trace elements that are found in one's body. The elements are at the same vibrational patterns that our bodies need to heal themselves. When this is over, if I have any ailments left, I will continue my study of crystal healing with a little bit of cookbook medicine. By matching up my problems with the recommended uses for each crystal listed on the various online stores, I will purchase my own crystals and see if I can fix what still needs fixin'. For the grand finale, I will track down the mystery of the crystal vortex, which draws funky people to Asheville like moths to a flame.

I am really getting into the groove of this "alternative medicine" thing. It seems like ages have passed since I thought naturopathy and chiropractic care were exotic. Crystals present a new frontier, at least from my perspective. I must remember that crystals have been the rage in certain circles since at least the 1960s.

Let the healing begin. I escape from work for another extended "lunch hour" to go on a "crystal journey with Michele." I have a lot of unanswered questions about crystal healing and, in particular, the John of God Crystal Bed. Who is this John of God? How does one become "of God?" Even Pope Francis isn't referred to as "Pope Francis of God." This John guy must have some powerful juju. What about the crystal bed? How does it work? If I stare at the crystals, will I burn my retina? These and other vexing questions beg to be answered. Hopefully, I will have the answers soon. I pull up to the Appalachian School of Holistic Herbalism. The school is located in an old, two-story house. Michele, an attractive middle-aged blond, garbed fully in white, meets me at the door. She guides me to her office on the second floor. The room is a repurposed single bedroom that now has two chairs, a side table, and the main attraction – a raised massage table with seven colored lights hanging over it.

The "crystal lights" are suspended over the bed by a pole with seven extendable arms. The walls are spartan with the exception of three framed 8" x 11" pictures: One is a picture of John of God, whom I recognize from Michele's website; the second is some unnamed saint (probably widely recognizable to most, but not to me); and the third is a pastel of a Buddha sitting cross-legged.

I take a seat across from Michele. We exchange a few pleasantries. She asks how I heard about the John of God Crystal Bed and what I hope to gain from the treatment. I respond, "I read about you during my online search of crystal therapies. I am intrigued by traditional Indian therapies." I tell her about my recent Ayurvedic experience. The tie between crystal therapy and traditional Hindu healing appears to be the recognition and manipulation of chakras – energy points on the body. She smiles approvingly. Michele then explains the Crystal Bed process. She suggests I limit my session to 30 minutes since I am a first-timer. "You never know how it will impact you," she says. She wants to be sure I am able drive myself back to work at the end of the session. I wonder what I am getting myself into. Are the lights really going to affect my sensorium? Perhaps the lights are really lasers that will be molding my body. What type of mind-altering experience have I signed up for? My heart rate increases.

I decide to ask a few more questions. "Who is John of God, and how is he related to the crystal bed?" Michele says that John of God is a spiritual healer famous for his paranormal healing ability. He has healed millions by acting as a conduit for spiritual entities, thus allowing him to perform both visible and invisible surgery. Michele visited John of God during a pilgrimage to Brazil. During her visit to his sanctuary, he identified her as someone with a gift for helping others. The John of God Crystal Bed provides a long-distance extension for his healing. As a "trance medium" and distance healer, he is able to cure people from far away. She encourages me to watch a video on her website, which shows an interview with Wayne Dyer on Oprah. Apparently, John of God successfully cured Mr. Dyer of leukemia, despite being a continent away. Michele says she is not exactly sure how he does it, but she has given up trying to find an explanation. "The results speak for themselves," she says. She tells me about a woman she treated for crippling arthritis, who, after a single crystal bed session, regained use of her arthritic hands. Others have reported sensing angels in the room while lying on the bed. For many, she says the impact is less dramatic, but most report a positive result, although it may be delayed for several days. It all sounds pretty impressive. I am ready to begin.

I lie fully clothed on the table. Michele lines up the seven crystal lights over each of my chakra points. She then covers my eyes with a towel and turns on soothing background music. She tells me to focus on one or two things I hope to achieve – these can be physical or mental. I choose to focus on becoming a better father – maintaining calm when dealing with my oldest son's quirks and compulsions, and being less overbearing with my middle son. I will let David determine his own fate in hockey. At times, I am too much of a "tiger dad," pushing my son too hard to excel. The second goal I choose is physical: I want to heal my bothersome left shoulder. I aggravated it while kayaking, and for the past several months, I have had to limit my athletic endeavors. Michele gives me a few moments to identify these goals, and after I acknowledge I have, she then has me take a few slow, deep breaths. She dims the lights and steps out of the room.

After lying still on the table for several minutes, and once I am relatively sure I am not being watched, curiosity gets the best of me. I lift the towel off my eyes and give the John of God Crystal Bed a closer look. The crystal lights appear to be little more than blinking plastic bulbs. They remind me of Christmas lights. I reach out and touch one – plastic, not warm, cheap. I do my inspection stealthily. What if Michele is observing my movements from outside the room and bursts in to expose me as a spy? I inspect the lights for a few more moments. With my curiosity satiated, I pull the towel back over my eyes, lie back, and enjoy an afternoon nap.

Thirty minutes later, Michele returns. She has me take a seat in one of the chairs, and she brings me a glass of water. She asks if I am okay to drive. "Yes," I say. She looks into my eyes to confirm that I am being truthful. After a few awkward moments, and after reassuring Michele that I have my wits about me, I write a check for $30 and make an exit.

What do I feel? Nothing . . . absolutely nothing. I certainly didn't sense any angels in the room or commune with John of God. Physically, I feel no different. This point is driven home when I reach across to adjust the tuner on my car CD player and feel the familiar twinge of pain in my shoulder. Was it a waste? It is too early to tell. I will give it the next couple of days to see if I appreciate any changes. I am not holding my breath while waiting for dramatic results. At the very least, a 30-minute siesta in the middle of a workday is always welcome and may be worth $30 in its own right. Although, if my prime desire is to take a noontime nap every day, I might as well move to Mexico.

If I need further proof my "John of God Crystal Bed" session was worthless, it comes later in the week – I am struck down by the flu. It is not just me, but the whole family who have become ill, the sole exception being my 13-year-old son Connor, who generally wants little to do with the rest of us. For once, his isolationism pays off. Why did we get sick? We don't deserve this. We are good people. We have been vaccinated. Apparently, the flu doesn't care. The predominant influenza strain circulating this year mutated just enough to make this year's flu vaccine relatively ineffective. Despite my diligently making sure everyone in the family was vaccinated, we have still been struck by a modern-day plague. I rarely miss work, but the flu has a way of changing one's tune. For the past three days, I have suffered muscle aches, headaches, chills, fever, and head congestion. To make matters worse, I haven't been able to hole up alone in my misery. Instead, the entire house reverberates with the sounds of coughing, sneezing and whining. This is an ideal time to escape to Asheville's Salt Cave.

Perhaps you are unaware that Asheville is a salt mining mecca . . . it is not. Always on the leading edge of the alternative movement, Asheville has one of a handful of artificially created salt caves in North America. The owners imported over twenty tons of Polish salt crystals to make their own cave. Why might one go to such lengths? Apparently, they take their cue from the Europeans, who have been basking in the benefits of "salt cave therapy" for decades. The Asheville Salt Cave claims to be an "alternative treatment" for a litany of conditions, including "acne, arthritis, asthma, bronchitis, migraines, viral infections, and weakened immune systems." I suffer from more than one of these maladies, and my immune system is certainly in a weakened state at the moment. A little spelunking in a salt cave is in order.

The Asheville Salt Cave is not dug into a remote mountain, but is smack dab in the middle of Asheville's bustling "business district." Rather than being overrun with big corporations, Asheville's downtown is an eclectic mix of restaurants, breweries, trinket shops, art galleries, and counter-culture establishments. The Salt Cave fits right in. The anteroom to the Salt Cave has a nice spa-vibe. There are Himalayan salt crystals of all sizes for sale, ranging from a few inches in diameter to the size of a football. After signing in, I am led to a long bench, which sits outside the closed entrance to the cave. I am encouraged to remove my shoes and to fix myself a cup of tea while waiting for my session to begin. The establishment is nice and cozy – a sharp contrast to the cold, drizzly weather outside. After a pleasant fifteen minutes of sipping herbal tea, I see the cave door open, and the attendant, a young woman in her twenties, invites us to come inside. I say "us," because I have been joined by a middle-aged Asheville woman of German descent.

As I enter the cave, I am struck by its appearance – it resembles the lower hold of an old two-masted ship. The entire "cave" is about 15 feet wide and 40 feet long. The walls are adorned with very large salt rocks that resemble stone masonry. The floor is covered with salt rock crystals of varying sizes on top of a virtual beach of sea salt. The ceiling has large wooden cross-ties holding up netting full of salt crystals the size of golf balls. In each corner is a fountain of flowing water, which adds to the ambiance and also aerosolizes the salt. Lights are set within some of the crystals on the wall and a few of the larger crystals on the ground. There are mats with pillows and blankets for lying on the sea salt-covered floor and anti-gravity lounge chairs for reclining. It is just like a day at the beach, except in a cave. The whole set-up reminds me of a *Star Trek* episode. I am in a cave on the planet Nubon, and the glowing salt crystals are alien eggs about to hatch.

The young attendant interrupts my intergalactic musings. She instructs us to find a comfortable place to relax, and I choose to lie on a floor mat. She tells us that the salt crystals, when heated to greater than 64 degrees (the room is about 70 degrees), release 84 trace elements and minerals necessary for our bodies. Breathing in these elements helps the body find balance and heal itself. We are also told the salt crystals neutralize the malicious positive ions that bombard us throughout the day. Positive ions are emitted by the electronics that are integral to life: cell phones, microwaves, computers, and televisions. In contrast, the Salt Cave releases negative ions to restore our balance. Negative ions reportedly have a wide range of beneficial effects from improved mood to better breathing. According to the attendant, "Forty-five minutes in the Salt Cave is equal to four days at the beach." As I lie back and grab a baseball-size salt crystal in my hand, I contemplate the healing that must have already begun.

Prior to leaving us to our own devices, our host guides us through some deep breathing and relaxation exercises. After she steps out, I begin to relax in earnest. We are in a dimly lit salt cave with gurgling fountains and soothing background music. This is a far cry from the hell my wife is currently experiencing at home. (I did invite my wife, but she claimed someone needed to watch over our feverish children – what a martyr.) The next 45 minutes pass quickly as I fade into my surroundings. As our time in the cave comes to an end, the lights brighten, and the door opens. After exiting and finding a seat on the wooden benches, I sip some more tea and pull on my shoes. The cost of this experience is a mere $15 – it is discount day for locals. Refreshed, I pull on my rain jacket and reenter the real world.

I return to work the following day. My fever has abated, and my congestion is less. Is the salt cave the reason? Perhaps . . . or could it be the Tamiflu (a prescription anti-viral) I started two days earlier?

To date, my exploration of crystal healing has been eye-opening, if not curative. With the aid of the John of God Crystal Bed and Asheville's Salt Cave, I am finally shrugging off the lingering effects of the flu. Hopefully, by relying on crystal magic once again, I can fight off the last remnants of this illness and tackle a few of my recurring complaints. I will now rely on some "cookbook medicine." Cookbook medicine is quite popular. It involves treating yourself by looking up your ailment in a book and then buying or making your own remedy, without the need of a doctor's prescription. This form of home brewing is also popular in homeopathy, herbal medicine, aromatherapy, and Appalachian medicine. My hope is to find a crystal that will cure my insomnia, tension headaches, and general laziness. The laziness to which I refer is my inclination to waste time surfing the Internet or checking my email for the hundredth time when I should be working on my book or doing some other task that is at least somewhat productive.

Before searching for my remedy, I will attempt to explain the theory behind how crystals work and define their role in curing various maladies. According to "reputable sources" (such as crystalwellbeing.co.uk), each "crystal has a unique internal structure, which causes it to resonate at a certain frequency. It is this resonance that is said to give crystals their healing abilities." The crystals help channel positive energy into the body, which promotes health and may cure disease. This gets a bit confusing if you consider I learned in the Salt Cave that positive ions emitted by electronics can cause imbalance and illness, which may in turn be reversed by the negative ions given off by crystals. The philosophy of crystal healing derives from Asian concepts such as life-energy (chi) and chakras. Remember the lines of chi which are stimulated during acupuncture? The chakras, otherwise referred to as vortices of energy, are said to connect the physical with the supernatural elements of the body. For each of the seven chakras on one's body, there is a corresponding color or crystal that can exert influence. (Now I understand the rationale behind the seven crystal lights that were aligned over my chakras during my John of God Crystal Bed Therapy.) Techniques may vary, but generally, one treats various ailments by picking the correct crystal for its corresponding chakra. Each chakra corresponds to an anatomical position on the body and not only exerts influence on particular organs or glands, but has further spiritual connections. The crystal is then laid over the chakra, dangled over the chakra, rubbed on the chakra, or just held near the chakra. Now that the "science" is all crystal clear, I am ready to heal myself.

I turn to the master cookbook – the Internet. I learn that the crown chakra (located just above one's head) and the brow chakra (located on the forehead) have influence over sleep patterns and headaches. The amethyst stone is the stone of choice for me. Apparently, the amethyst is a pretty powerful stone. It is commonly used as a "dream stone" to help with insomnia, and it can relieve headaches by being rubbed across one's forehead. Better yet, it is said to promote mental clarity. When the amethyst is placed on the crown chakra, it encourages positive thought patterns and exerts control over the pineal gland. In medical school, we learned that the pineal gland secretes melatonin, which affects our sleep-wake cycles. The brow chakra exerts influence over the pituitary gland, which is a principle regulator of our endocrine system. Amethyst crystals are noted to have several other properties: they improve memory, protect from danger, and are thought to bring success in business. This stone sure has some powerful mojo. After completing my amethyst education, I tell my wife I need to take a trip to the crystal shop (we have several in Asheville) so that I can buy myself a stone. Always a step ahead of me, she gives a knowing smile and asks if I might be able to hold off until after Christmas. When I say "no," she goes to our bedroom and returns holding a small package. "Since you can't wait," she says. I rip open the package and lo and behold, sitting inside the box are two amethysts – a small one to carry in my pocket and a larger cluster of crystals for my bedside. How did she know I was planning on buying these? I am not sure . . . woman's intuition or crystal magic?

Over the following week, I dutifully carry the smaller amethyst in my pocket throughout the day. At night, before going to sleep, I place the larger crystal over both my crown and brow chakras. Just before drifting off to sleep, I slip the large crystal under my pillow. As I close my eyes, I imagine healing ions flowing through my body as I am transmuted to a higher plane. At the end of the week, I take stock of my condition. Has the amethyst lived up to its billing? Despite some remaining head congestion, I have been sleeping well, and I have been headache free all week. I am not sure if I have achieved full mental clarity, but I have been more motivated to write during my free time. Perhaps more significantly, I made a rare good financial decision (I suggest this qualifies as "business success"): I rebalanced my retirement portfolio to an increased weight in stocks just before the stock market rallied. This is a sharp contrast with the normal Mahan philosophy of buy high, sell low. I am not sure Janet Yellen's economic statements can be attributed to the amethyst, but who knows.

Taking stock of my crystal experience so far: perhaps the crystals work after all. I did manage to avoid getting as sick as my wife during our recent flu bout, and I have recovered faster. One might look at her as the control in my study of crystals. We both got sick around the same time, but only I experienced the Salt Cave and slept with an amethyst under my pillow. If this is not definitive proof, I don't know what is. At the very least, therapy with crystals has little downside; they are easy to use and they have few side-effects . . . except for a lumpy pillow.

Weeks have passed. I have been trying to carve out a weekend day for my final crystal adventure. During this last stage of my investigation into the magic of crystals, I will be graduating from hand-held crystals to crystals of a much bigger magnitude. What am I talking about? I am referring to the unique crystal lattice structure that undergirds the western North Carolina mountains. This crystal lattice is believed to contribute to multiple energy vortices in the region. The largest of these energy vortices is said to be Mount Mitchell, the highest mountain east of the Mississippi River. New Age devotees claim Mt. Mitchell is at the intersection of several ley lines (intersections which connect places of geographical and historical significance). This intersection of energy is felt to be the source of a huge fount of energy, or vortex. Some even claim these vortices channel extraterrestrial cosmic energy. This influx of cosmic and spiritual energy creates a special vibe in Asheville, which attracts "certain" kinds of people. This might explain the interesting nexus of personalities in the region, ranging from the highly religious to the earthy spiritual types. I certainly have had no problems finding believers of every type in Asheville. Up until now, I attributed my improvement in sleep and a more relaxed attitude to my new job and living in a beautiful setting. Perhaps my perception is flawed. Instead, it is the cosmic energy infusing this region that that has improved my mental outlook.

With this new understanding, I decide the cherry on the sundae of my crystal investigations will be to go to the power center itself, the peak of Mount Mitchell. I hoped to bike from my house to the summit, but I am not in great shape at the moment, and I don't have five or more hours to spare. Instead, I load my bike into the back of my Honda Civic, and I head for the base of the mountain. My drive gets off to a great start. A mere 200 yards from my house, I encounter a juvenile black bear crossing the road. Seeing wildlife always puts me in a good mood. With the windows down and music playing, I drive towards Mount Mitchell on the Blue Ridge Parkway. This is a beautiful drive. The trees all have their new spring leaves, and the roadside flowers are in bloom.

I can't help but feel relaxed and happy as I wind my way through the mountains. I feel a bit guilty as I pass cyclists laboring up the Parkway. The summit of Mount Mitchell is likely the goal for many of them. I, on the other hand, drive to the Mount Mitchell Park entrance, pull to the side of the road, and unload my bike. I quickly hop on my bike and leave my car behind. If any fellow cyclists see me, they will probably tell me I am cheating. It is only a little over three miles from the park entrance to the summit, but it is a hardy climb nonetheless.

The climb is steep, but it is gorgeous. The roadside is covered with wildflowers. As I climb higher, I can smell the pine trees and see birds flittering among the treetops. I pass one biker who is walking his bike. I guiltily speed by on my fresh legs. He is probably impressed with my stamina. Finally, I arrive at the uppermost parking lot. From here, I must walk my bike the last 300 or so yards from the visitor center to the summit. At the summit, I pose for a picture – not a selfie, but a photo taken by someone else. I then walk to a raised platform that has overlooks for 360 degrees. It is stunning. I can see towards Asheville, from whence I came. I can see towards Tennessee, Virginia, and the distant Atlantic coast. I can almost feel the energy emanating from the center of the mountain and rising up through my feet. After communing with nature for twenty or so minutes, I walk back down to the visitor center and begin the refreshing coast down the mountain to my car.

As I drive back home with a smile on my face, I contemplate the idea of energy vortices. It all seems a bit far-fetched. More likely, it is the natural beauty of the area that draws people rather than a cosmic force, but who am I to question? I certainly feel energized and will be drawn back to this area again and again. It is either just a great place to live, or little green men have a plan for me.

## Crystal Therapy

**<u>Cost</u>:**

**Crystal Bed Therapy** – $20/session

**Salt Cave** – $15-30/session

**Do-it-yourself crystals** – $5-$100/crystal

**Energy Vortex** – Free (or "priceless" as they say in the MasterCard commercials)

**Covered by standard insurance policies:** No

**Published research:**

Presentation at Sixth European Congress of Psychology in Rome, 1999 ("Crystal clear: paranormal powers, placebo, or priming?") concluded no benefit of crystals.[1]

Same study replicated by O'Donnell, H., and Williams, L., presented to the British Psychological Society Centary Annual Conference in Glasgow in 2001 (this time double-blinded) yielded same results – no benefit.[2]

# Endnotes

1 French, C. C., & Williams, L. (1999). Crystal clear: paranormal powers, placebo, or priming? Sixth European Congress of Psychology, Rome, 4-9 July 1999.

2 French, C. C., O'Donnell, H., & Williams, L. (2001). Hypnotic susceptibility, paranormal belief and reports of 'crystal power.' British Psychological Society Centenary Annual Conference, Glasgow, 28-31 March 2001. (Abstract published in *Proceedings of the British Psychological Society,* 9(2), 186).

# Chapter 18 Fifteen-Yard Penalty for Roughing – Rolfing

This chapter was never meant to be. After five years of exploring alternative therapies, I formed a pretty good idea of what is "alternative" and what is not. Most forms of massage are not alternative, or so I thought. In my mind, Rolfing is just another form of deep-tissue massage, and what is alternative about deep-tissue massage? My impression is that most professional athletes get deep-tissue massages on a daily basis. I don't imagine LeBron James embraces alternative medicine, but I could be wrong. My father, a retired physician, is a Rolfing devotee. Like me, he suffers from chronic lower back pain. He swears that Rolfing raised him from the dead. For several years, he has encouraged me to try Rolfing and has sent me newspaper articles about the miracles of Rolfing. Typical of all offspring, I am reluctant to follow the advice of my parent. In truth, my reasons for not trying Rolfing are fourfold. First, it is expensive – about $100 a session. Second, to do it right, the whole Rolfing experience takes much longer than the allotted one month that I have spent on the majority of my explorations. Third, it looks painful. Some call it "massage for masochists." My prior experience with "deep-tissue massage," the closest thing I can equate to Rolfing, is seared into my memory. I recall a woman pressing so hard and deep into my lower abdomen that I thought my appendix would rupture. Last, is it really alternative medicine if my dad is doing it?

What changed my mind? I planned a return trip to Ghana to see my friend Edmund and to give a few medical lectures to the residents at the university where he works. I put a lot of work into preparing for this trip. I spent days preparing lectures, arranging my itinerary, applying for a visa, and getting the required pre-travel vaccinations and anti-malarial pills. With the day of departure fast approaching, disaster struck. One week before my scheduled overnight flight to Ghana, excruciating back pain woke me up in the middle of the night. My back acts up about once every year or two. The timing could not have been worse. Usually an episode cripples me for four to six weeks. The first two weeks, I am severely limited in my activity and forced to spend as much time as possible lying on the ground with my feet propped up in the air. I envision the overnight flight in the coach section followed by arriving in the chaos of West Africa. This will be followed by hours standing on my feet giving lectures and doing medical rounds. Lying on my back in an air-conditioned room is a pipe dream. It is not a pretty picture. I really want to go on this trip. The last time I was in Ghana was 1998, and I have been looking forward to returning ever since. I am desperate. I am willing to try anything that might make me travel worthy.

When I hobble into work on Monday, five days before my planned departure, I arouse the empathy of my officemate, Jim Satterly. Jim is a hospitalist who covers the nightshift. He works every other week and goes home at 8 a.m., just as I am arriving. Despite sharing an office, our paths cross for only a short period every other week. Jim is a great guy. I think he prefers working the nightshift because the hospital is quieter, and he can avoid the office politics that occur during the daytime. He went to an osteopathic medical school, whereas I went to an allopathic one. The difference is that osteopaths, in addition to basic medical training, are instructed in manipulating the spine and skeleton, similar in some ways to chiropractors, while allopathic doctors are not. As a hospitalist in a Veterans Hospital, Jim rarely gets an opportunity to employ the manipulation component of his training. Seeing my obvious discomfort and eager to employ his rarely used skills of spinal manipulation, Jim offers to perform a few adjustments to my spine and pelvis on the floor of our office. With the door locked, of course, Jim assesses me while I stand and then bend over at the waist. He has me lie down on the floor and performs some adjustments to my legs and pelvis. He does this on each of the next two mornings when our shifts overlap. Despite his ministrations, after a couple of days, I don't feel much difference. In fairness to Jim, our office floor is not the perfect condition for his work. Jim can sense my frustration, and he is aware that the date of my departure is looming. Rather than give up hope, he recommends I see a Rolfer. Jim has had issues with his own back and joints, and he believes a good Rolfing is just what I need. Desperate times call for desperate measures.

There are a plethora of Rolfers in Asheville, further bolstering my opinion that Rolfing is not truly alternative. How do I choose? Groupon, of course. I schedule a visit for the following day. Despite Jim's adjustments of my back, I am still an invalid, and my trip to Ghana is now only a couple of days away. I arrive at the Rolfer with high expectations. I look forward to some deep massage on my back. I am willing to put up with some discomfort, even pain, during the massage if I am able to walk upright again as a result. I meet the Rolfer and sheepishly admit I am using a Groupon for my visit, but he is unperturbed. I am ready to get down to business. The Rolfer, on the other hand, is in no rush. He spends the next 45 minutes explaining the theory of Rolfing. Can't he see my discomfort? Sitting in a hard, straight-backed chair, I am very uncomfortable. He is oblivious as he excitedly explains why I am having pain. He uses a taut string model to explain a concept he calls "tensegrity." Apparently, the various strings represent the fascia of my body. When the fascia, the fibrous tissue that envelopes our muscles and tissues, falls out of balance, the entire framework of our body goes out of whack, and we are prone to aches and injury.

After an extensive demonstration, he finally recognizes my discomfort (perhaps it is the sweat on my brow or my periodic moans) and has me lie down on the massage table. He spends the next hour giving me a deep massage with a focus on my back. I wince at times as he drives his fist and elbows into my back, but overall, it is tolerable. He definitely works out the kinks in my back. As I drive home that afternoon, my back feels much better. I am able to walk upright. Perhaps I will be going to Ghana after all. Unfortunately, over the course of the next day, my back pain recurs with a vengeance. I am forced to cancel my trip the morning of my planned departure. Although I don't make my trip, my brief exposure to Rolfing makes me realize it is as "alternative" as any other therapy I have experienced. I decide I will give Rolfing a real try, but with a Rolfer who doesn't talk so much.

To learn more about Rolfing, I go straight to what should be the definitive source, the website of the Rolf Institute of Structural Integration. Rolfing is named after its founder, Dr. Ida Rolf. Dr. Rolf began teaching Structural Integration in the 1950s, and she founded the Rolf Institute of Structural Integration in 1971. "Rolfing Structural Integration is a form of bodywork that reorganizes the connective tissues, called fascia, that permeates the entire body."[1] Dr. Rolf, a biochemist by training, observed that the body is seamlessly connected by the fascia, which must be properly aligned or the body will fall out of balance. When the fascia becomes rigid and sticky, it can restrict the movement of muscles and joints. Practitioners of Structural Integration, or Rolfing, use pressure applied with their fingers, fists, and elbows to release fascial adhesions. According to my bible of alternative medicine, "pain may be felt when pressure is applied."

Dr. Rolf said that to make profound tissue changes, one could hardly expect this to be accomplished without a "dramatic reaction."[2] I presume she means pain. The typical "recipe," as it is sometimes called, is a progression of ten sessions, which allow a systematic approach to improve alignment and movement of the body. It sounds like a good gimmick to ensure return business. According to the Rolfing website, over 1 million people have received Rolfing work. Based on my informal survey of Ashevillians, the number is probably much higher.

My proposed trip to Ghana is now long passed, my severe back pain has abated, and I finally arrange an appointment with a new Rolfer. I am going to give "the recipe" a try. This time, I abandon Groupon and choose a Rolfer who practices in downtown Asheville. His office is located in a very old structure that appears to have once been a house. As I step into the foyer, I smell incense wafting through the air. Based upon the placards on the doors and the calling cards on the entry table, it appears that every office space in the building houses a practitioner of alternative therapy – masseuses, naturopaths, etc. I climb a staircase to the second floor and knock on the door of my Rolfer. John opens the door and leads me into an expansive room with a high ceiling and a massage table in the center. There is soothing background music playing and a few nature photos on the wall. The room is airy, but still warm and comforting. I am surprised to see that John appears to be my reflection. He is my height, just over six feet tall, has blond hair, and has my build. He is conservatively dressed with a short-sleeved knit shirt and khaki pants. Perhaps the main distinction between us is that he is barefoot. He certainly does not fit my preconceived notion of an alternative practitioner.

At John's direction, I sit in a chair along the wall. He sits across from me on the edge of the massage table. He then launches into the theory of Rolfing. Instead of the tensegrity model, he has a two-foot tall model skeleton, which he uses to explain the connectivity and role of the fascia. He stresses that the goal of Rolfing is to undo restrictions in the fascia in order to open up space, thereby allowing the muscles and skeleton to return to their normal balanced positions. He recommends ten sessions so that he can systematically work on my entire fascial system. Mercifully, the entire explanation takes only 15 minutes. I like this guy. Time to begin.

I disrobe down to my boxers. John observes me standing and walking. I then lie down on the massage table, and he covers me with a thin blanket. He goes to work on my forearm, upper arms, and chest. He uses his fingers, knuckles, and even his elbows depending on how much pressure he wants to apply. The sensation varies from intense to downright painful. He periodically asks if he is pressing too hard. I invariably answer "no" for fear of diminishing the experience. While working on my shoulders and chest, he uses his whole body weight while digging his elbows between my strands of muscles. Over the course of the first session, he also works on my outer thighs and buttocks. The amount of pressure he applies over my larger muscle groups is severe. Sweat forms on my brow. Ouch. While working on my thighs, he instructs me to "breathe into my pelvis." I try to breathe into my pelvis, but actually I am just rocking my pelvis while taking a deep breath. If my recollection of anatomy is correct, my lungs do not extend anywhere near my pelvis, but who am I to question? My rocking of the pelvis seems to satisfy John. Periodically, John takes a pause from Rolfing, apparently as much to give him a break as me. He also has me stand up so he can again observe me standing and walking. He solicits my observations regarding how I feel after each major segment of my body has been worked on. After manipulating the right side of my chest, he asks how

I feel. He tells me to compare the feeling in the two sides of my body. I say that the right side of my chest feels more open – less restrictive, my breathing discordant. He likes this response. John is very pleasant, and when not instructing me in breathing techniques or telling me to flex a particular muscle group, he keeps up a pleasant banter about all aspects about my life and his. We have a lot in common.

Later in the first session, he digs his fist into the front of my neck while I am lying flat on my back. He presses deeply next to my larynx, my breathing tube. I am fearful he will rupture the cartilage in my larynx. I am relieved when he finishes this maneuver, and I can still breathe. He finishes the session by having me sit on a stool while he works on my abdomen and back. At the end of session, he encourages me to observe how I feel throughout the week. I write him a check for $120 and schedule session number two for the following week.

Escaping from work during the hours he is available is tricky. I shoot for the late afternoon times when I will have, hopefully, finished my day's work. It feels a bit risky to turn off my cell phone and pager at four o'clock in the afternoon. It is a bit irresponsible of me, considering I am the only infectious disease physician at my hospital. Nevertheless, two hours outside the grasp of medical colleagues and patients feels decadent, maybe the most relaxing component of the whole endeavor. At the end of the first session, I nervously turn my pager and cell phone back on to see if there are any frantic messages. Fortunately, my services were not needed during session one.

The next day, my body feels unrestricted. My rib cage feels open and more expansive than normal. I am not sure if these sensations are real or just thoughts planted by my Rolfer. My chest muscles are sore where he drove his elbow into them, but overall I feel pretty good. He told me the next session would focus primarily on my lower extremities, particularly my feet. Just the mention of touching my feet makes me afraid, very afraid. My feet, particularly the bottoms of my feet, are very sensitive. I am not sure I will be able to tolerate it. We will see.

All too quickly, my second Rolfing session rolls around. Overall, the second session is similar to the first. He assesses my standing, my gait, and asks me how I feel between working on various sections of my body. This time, however, he gives particular attention to my feet. I always feel like a little kid when someone touches my feet. They are so sensitive that my initial reaction is to quickly pull them away and start laughing. I steel my nerves for the inevitable. Amazingly, I allow him to touch the bottom of my feet without any violent response on my part. Quickly, I realize that being tickled is not what I should have feared. Pain is a more apt description. He uses his knuckles and even his forearm to work the knots out of the fascia on the bottoms of my feet. As he begins to press, I only feel pressure, but the sensation builds to an almost unbearable climax as he sustains the pressure while working on the knotted fascia. I have a history of plantar fasciitis, so maybe he is breaking up some serious scar tissue. It is almost more than I can handle. Just when I am about to scream, he lets up. Later in the session, he has me sit up on the edge of the massage table with my feet flat on the floor. He then pulls up a chair facing me and uses his feet to massage the tops of mine. We are playing footsies. This feels very intimate. I half expect him to lean over and give me a kiss, but he does not.

After working on my feet, he again assesses my gait and asks me how I feel. My initial thought is that I survived the torture chamber, but then I channel my inner Buddha and determine how I really feel. My feet feel great. They feel flat. Not bad flat, but good flat. It is as if all the tension in my feet has been expunged, and my foot muscles are finally relaxed enough to appreciate the earth again. I am euphoric, having survived the foot phase of Rolfing, but I also appreciate the potential benefits. He instructs me to walk barefoot as much as possible in the coming days. I do. For several days, I am more in tune to how my feet feel. Shod or unshod, my feet feel pretty good.

Over the following weeks, I continue to see John about once a week. Occasionally, we are unable to find a time that agrees with both of our schedules, and the next visit is put off a week or two, but he is unconcerned. Throughout these visits, a pattern is established – he observes my posture and my walk, both at the beginning and periodically throughout each session while always eliciting feedback regarding how I feel. I have learned the lingo that makes the Rolfer happy – "I feel looser," "less restricted," "open," and "more free." Again, I am not always sure I believe what I am saying, but at times I am convinced. He works my whole body in the first few sessions, and then in sessions four through seven, he focuses on my core. I find the notion of working on the fascia surrounding my anterior spine via my abdomen a bit disconcerting. I flashback to my experience with deep-tissue massage, and I remember feeling that my inner organs will rupture. He uses his hands to work deep into my abdomen. He says he is creating suction with his palms and thereby influencing the deeper tissues. I am not sure about the suction, but his hands are digging much deeper than seems appropriate.

Throughout each session, we keep a healthy banter going. In addition to discussing the more mundane components of our lives, he opens up to me regarding the alternative medicine community. In a rare instance of openness, I reveal that I am writing a book about my alternative medicine experience. I usually keep this secret for fear that people will treat me differently, perhaps seeing me as a skeptic. He is nonplussed. In fact, I think this has led him to open up to me even more than he otherwise might. John is definitely a true believer. He says that although he was schooled in the art of Rolfing, it wasn't until he began practicing Rolfing that he became convinced of its benefits. He has seen his clients transformed by "the recipe." He goes to a Rolfer himself and attests to the benefits of periodically going back for a series of sessions. I not only probe his knowledge of Rolfing, but I inquire about his opinion of other forms of alternative medicine. Interestingly, he is acquainted with my naturopath and also seems to have at least a casual friendship with Mark Hymen, the author of the UltraSimple Diet. John agrees with the hypothesis of "inflammation" being a root cause for many of our health problems. My discussion with John leaves me even more convinced that "alternative medicine" is a way of life rather than a single discipline. There are several common themes adopted by all walks of alternative medicine: inflammation, connectiveness, chakras, and balance are terms that recur although the term "tensegrity," which seems to be made-up, is unique to Rolfing.

Not only does John provide me with insight into the alternative medicine culture, but our discussions are strangely therapeutic. One commonality among alternative practitioners is that they never seem rushed. As opposed to a Western doctor, who might be seeing 20 patients a day for 15 minutes each, my experience with alternative practitioners is just the opposite. They seem to have a less hectic schedule and are willing to take the time to listen to you, all of which contributes to a feeling of calm. My sessions with John are long, unrushed, and therapeutic on many levels. I am not sure if I derive more benefit from the talking or the Rolfing. Once a week, I escape to John's enclave, I turn off my pager and cell phone, and I relax – or sort of relax when I am not having an elbow driven into my thigh. I have a lot of stressors in my life. A 90-minute break from the pressures of the world where all I need to focus on is whether my fascia is too tight is pretty special. John and I talk about our families, work, and anything else that comes to mind. It is sad to say, but I have opened up more to John than any other person in Asheville, aside from my wife. I find developing close male bonds difficult as an adult; perhaps this is why so many adults see a therapist, a hired confidant.

Finally, session six rolls around. It is time to focus on the lower back. This is the session I have been waiting for. He thoroughly works on my calves, buttocks, pelvis, and lower back. Despite being the "lower back" session, I am disappointed more time is not spent actually pressing over my lower back. I remind myself it is all about "creating space" to allow my back muscles and spine to move back into their proper alignment. After working on my pelvis, he observes me walk. He comments on the swing of my hips. He says that after opening my pelvis, my hips should sway so that I might feel like I am walking like a woman – hmmm . . . not so sure about that.

Subsequent to the session on my lower back, I take stock of my general well-being. Over the next week, I am able to do activities pain-free that I normally would not attempt. My wife's brother and his children come to visit, and we play soccer. I find myself sprinting up and down the field with no limitation. In fact, I actually race my 15-year-old nephew in a sprint, and I don't pull my hamstring. I haven't opened it up like that in years. Later in the week, I go mountain biking – no pain, and I even shoot hockey in the basement with my son and feel no pain in my chronically inflamed shoulder. What is going on? Could this Rolfing actually be working?

I eagerly attend session seven, which focuses on my upper spine and head. I am eager for this session – nothing like a relaxing neck massage. Perhaps I will become so relaxed I will fall asleep during this session. Quickly, I realize sleep is a fantasy. John works on my shoulders, my upper chest, and the front of my neck. Again, as he digs his fist into my neck, I fear he may rupture my larynx. Then things turn strange. John places little plastic covers on his fingers and starts to massage my gums – not just my outer gum line as a dentist might do, but my inner gums and deep into my mouth. I do my best not to gag. I have a hard time reconciling the purpose of this oral maneuver. Is there really restrictive fascia in my mouth? When the session is complete, will my teeth and jaw be free to move into "proper alignment." Could this this be a cheaper alternative to braces? Needless to say, I am relieved when the oral probing is complete. I have survived the worst . . . or have I? Now things become even weirder.

John removes the finger covers from his index fingers and, to my amazement, places two new plastic finger covers on each of his pinkies. I contemplate cutting the session short. Perhaps I should feign an emergency. Alas, both my pager and my cell phone are turned off. There is no chance for respite. I eye John warily as he approaches the head of the massage table. The next thing I know, both his pinkies are deep into my nostrils. I want to yell, "Mercy!" The only thing that keeps me quiet is the realization that this will be a juicy tidbit for my book. He spends the next five minutes probing the inner recesses of my nasal cavity. My nose has never been probed so deeply, even as a child. I am incredulous. This truly puts the "alternative" into alternative medicine. I mention to John that we scold our son Thayer for picking his nose, but perhaps he is just practicing to become a Rolfer; John laughs. Again, I wonder what fascia is restricted in my nose. Will my nose be straighter once we are done? Finally, the probing comes to a merciful end. I hope he doesn't ask me if my mouth and nose feel less restricted. For the next week, my nose just feels funny – like it has been violated. Nose abuse.

The last three sessions are all about consolidation. Similar to sessions one through three, John works me from top to bottom. During one of these sessions, when he is again using his entire body weight to dig his elbow into my leg and then my chest, it crosses my mind that perhaps this could actually be harmful. Could he be injuring me? Could one develop rhabdomyolysis (muscle injury leading to release of muscle enzymes that can be harmful to one's kidneys) from Rolfing? I do my best to suppress these thoughts. In our tenth and final session, he has me stand and asks me to imagine a line running down through the center of my body pulling me straight and upright. He watches my gait. I feel taller. He smiles. He says I appear more balanced and my gait is improved. He comments that I should continue to further appreciate the benefits of the Rolfing sessions for months to come, as my muscles and skeleton continue to move into proper alignment via the space that has been created.

Parting is bittersweet. Overall, I enjoyed my Rolfing experience. I enjoyed the long escapes from work, the less painful parts of the Rolfing, and making a new friend. I managed to pull this off without getting fired from work (the long absences with my pager and cell phone off could have created some problems, but didn't). I won't miss the expense. Although $120 for a 90-minute session may not seem like much, it does start to add up over time. John suggests that in a few months, I might derive additional benefit by returning for a series of three more sessions and then periodically thereafter. We will see.

What is my assessment of Rolfing? I honestly became more skeptical as I got further into the "recipe." The exploration of my mouth and nasal cavity seems without basis. Some of the deep probing with his elbow might have been more harmful than good. I harken back to Ida Rolf's statement that discomfort may be felt when pressure is applied, but "people often call this reaction pain, but it is not the pain with associate injury or hurt." So she says. I did find one published case of significant muscle injury with resultant kidney failure attributed to massage[3]; based on my search I would say rhabdomyolysis due to Rolfing is possible, but extremely unlikely. On the plus side, I did have a sense of "openness" of my musculature in the days after each session, and I was able to perform some activities pain-free which I had not done for a long time. Will the benefits last? For me, the answer seems to be "no." Over the next couple of weeks, my shoulder pain returns and I again wrench my back. I do pay more attention to my posture. I try not to slump in my chair at work. Aside from these benefits, I am unconvinced. The Rolfing "recipe" took a lot of time and money with little clear long-term gain, but I did enjoy the psychotherapy.

## Rolfing (Structural Integration)

**Cost: $100-$150/ 90-minute session**

**Covered by standard insurance policies:** No

**Published research:**

An extensive review published in 2004 found insufficient evidence that Rolfing is effective for the treatment of any health condition.[4]

A 1979 study evaluated the effects of Rolfing on 48 patients with anxiety. After five weeks of treatment, patients who received Rolfing therapy experienced a greater decrease in anxiety than those in a control group. This was measured by questionnaires administered to all of the subjects before and after the five-week study, which focused on release of emotional tension stored in muscles.[5]

A 2006 Cochrane Database Review of studies evaluating the efficacy of manual therapies in reducing pain from tension-type headache (TTH) found two trials involving connective tissue manipulation and one trial using soft-tissue massage. Both techniques showed limited evidence of effectiveness in reducing pain from TTH.[6]

There are several other smaller, non-controlled studies, which have had inconclusive results.

# Endnotes


1 http://www.rolf.org/about. Accessed 7/13/2015.

2 Trivieri, L. & Anderson, J.W. *Alternative medicine – the definitive guide* (2nd ed.). Ten Speed Press. 2002.

3 Lai, M.Y., et al. Fever with acute renal failure due to body massage-induced rhabdomyolysis. *Nephrol. Dial. Transplant*, 2006. 21(1): 233-234.

4 Jones, T.A. (2004). Rolfing. *Physical Medicine and Rehabilitation Clinics of North America*, 15(4):799–809.

5 Weinberg, R.S. & Hunt, V.V. Effects of structural integration on state-trait anxiety. *J Clin Psychol*, 1979 Apr;35(2):319-22.

6 Fernandez-de-Las-PeÃas, C., Alonso-Blanco, C, Cuadrado, M.L., et al. Are manual therapies effective in reducing pain from tension-type headache?: a systematic review. *Clin J Pain,* 2006 Mar-Apr;22(3): 278-85.

# Chapter 19 Craniosacral Therapy – Molding the Mind

I began my exploration of alternative medicine five years ago. For my final experience, I will try craniosacral therapy (CST). It is fitting that I wrap up my adventures with craniosacral therapy because, if you remember, it was my wife's reaction to Andrew Weil's description of CST that spurred me to begin this quest. Beth read me the account of a craniosacral practitioner who claimed to feel the movement of the skull bones as a means to diagnosis and treat health problems. I was in disbelief: "The movements of the skull bones?!" Beth, on the other hand, thought the explanation was perfectly reasonable. Despite my inherent skepticism to CST, who was I to contradict the author's testimony? I might be a physician, but I never tried CST myself, nor do I have any proof that it doesn't work. It just sounds kooky. Our discussion of CST led me to consider the entire field of alternative medicine. My Western training told me it was all kooky, but I also realized my opinion was based on biases formed in my training in traditional Western medicine. Rather than disparage alternative medicine while being uninformed, I decided to give it a try and develop my own educated opinion. Here I am, five years into my alternative education, and I have come full circle. I will undergo CST. I am certainly much more open-minded, but I still have a hard time imagining my skull bones being free-floating.

I assume finding a craniosacral therapist will be difficult, but once again Asheville's deep well of alternative medicine practitioners comes through. In fact, the CST business appears to be booming – I have multiple options to choose from. CST is performed by massage therapists, practitioners of holistic healing, chiropractors, and others, although the massage therapists seem to be the most numerous. I choose a husband-wife team who are both licensed massage therapists. In addition to CST, they offer reflexology and more traditional forms of massage. According to their website, the craniosacral system consists of the protective membranes surrounding the brain, the lining of the cranium, and the covering of the spinal column, as well as the cerebrospinal fluid, which ebbs and flows at a rate of six to ten cycles per minute. The cerebrospinal fluid represents the body's hydraulic system and also supports the entire nervous system. Events ranging from a traumatic birth to other physical and emotional traumas occurring later in life can upset the rhythms of these systems.

The website explains that CST follows a gentle, light-pressure protocol to enhance the body's natural ability to heal, improve brain and spinal cord function, and restore immune system response. Some of the maladies that CST claims to heal are migraine headaches, TMJ (temporomandibular joint pain), chronic neck and shoulder pain, fibromyalgia, emotional difficulties, learning disabilities, and joint and muscle pain. This seems perfect for me. Despite my recent Rolfing experience, I still have lower back pain, and I am prone to frequent headaches.

My alternative medicine bible reiterates the claimed benefits of CST touted by the website.[1] In fact, it expands the range of problems that can be addressed to include respiratory conditions, digestive disorders, and even Down syndrome. A cranial therapist is trained to feel the motion of the craniosacral system and locate critical points of restriction, which can then be manipulated to re-establish a normal rhythm. There are three primary approaches to CST: the sutural approach, the meningeal approach, and the reflex approach. The pioneers of CST are Dr. William Sutherland in the early 20$^{th}$ century and later Dr. John Upledger in the 1970s, both osteopathic physicians. Dr. Sutherland popularized the sutural approach in which he manipulated the sutures (where the cranial bones meet) to increase the mobility of the cranial bones. This approach is interesting, but I am instantly skeptical. I learned early in my medical training to palpate the cranium of infants for their fontanelles, or "soft spots," during the first year of life as a possible indication of their volume status (level of hydration). There are two main soft spots, one at the front of the skull and one near the back. When an infant is dehydrated or sick, the fontanelles may be sunken in. These spots represent the areas where the cranial sutures have yet to fuse. Early on, the cranial bones are unfused to allow the brain room to grow. By 12-18 months of age, the cranial bones have fused – the lines of fusion are called the suture lines. Once the cranial bones fuse, I doubt much movement could be appreciated. Harkening back to my first year of medical school when I dissected a cadaver in gross anatomy, I remember palpating these very same suture lines and appreciating the skull as a single fused structure.

Dr. Upledger built upon Dr. Sutherland's approach and pioneered the meningeal approach. Dr. Upledger claimed this approach was very successful for treating chronic, severe headaches. His approach, which happens to be the approach followed by the massage therapist I will be seeing, works on releasing the restrictions of the cranial tissues and underlying membranes while monitoring the rhythmic movement of the craniosacral system via changes in cerebrospinal fluid pressure. Dr. Upledger reported an 85% success rate in curing headaches. My headaches are feeling better already. I book a visit for the following week.

My appointment finally comes around. I am able to book a 5 p.m. appointment, so for once I am able to leave my work at my normal time and not have to sneak out early while pursuing my "alternative" endeavors. The office is located on a trendy street in North Asheville not far from the Grove Park Inn, a famous resort. The massage therapist's office is located in an older single-story cottage. I am met at the door by the therapist, a middle-aged woman with a warm smile. After exchanging pleasantries, she escorts me into the outer vestibule. Here, I take a seat and fill out the requisite forms: who am I, what is my profession, next of kin, how did I hear of them, and what am I here for today? Throughout my exploration of alternative medicine, I often waffle on how to answer this second question – what is my profession? I don't like to lie, but I also don't want to be too truthful. Perhaps if they know I am a medical doctor, they will treat me differently and cheat me out of some of the alternative experience. I signify that I am a "writer," hoping this will not lead to a host of difficult questions: "What have you authored?" "Have I read any of your works?" Fortunately, when reading the form, she says, "A writer, hmm . . . you must be hunched over a computer quite a lot," to which I say, "yes." And then she moves on to other things. My alias is not blown. I tell her about my headaches and back pain, and she smiles and tells me that CST should be just the thing to help me feel better.

Next the therapist leads me into an octagonal room with a massage table in the center. It smells of incense (the calling card of alternative practitioners). The room has carpeted floors and dark wood walls. There is a lava lamp (yes, they still do exist) sitting on a side table. There is a framed illustration of a man and a woman with their muscles and skeleton exposed. Also included on the diagram are labeled acupoints and lines of meridian – another commonality that spans several alternative disciplines, including massage, crystal therapy, and acupuncture. Soothing music plays in the background; it sounds like a didgeridoo from Australia. I succumb to the moment. Let the healing begin.

I remain fully dressed and lie face up on the massage table. The therapist's hands meticulously feel along my scalp, apparently palpating the suture lines between my cranial bones. I wonder if she can feel subtle movements of my cranial bones or perhaps even deeper movements in my brain. She then places her hands at the base of my skull in the back of my neck, where I imagine she is feeling for cerebrospinal fluid (CSF) pulsations. She jams her thumbs into this area at the base of my skull while encouraging me to relax my head back. It is not the most relaxing position, but I try to channel my inner Buddha. After a few minutes, she moves to the foot of the table and pulls gently on my feet and applies pressure with her hands over my knees, thighs, pelvis, chest, and shoulders. She then returns to the base of my skull for a while. During the course of the visit, she spends time pressing gently along my skull, ears and face. Fortunately, she does not enter my nose – I have had enough of the inner nose manipulation by my Rolfer. Periodically, she reassesses the rhythm of my CSF by probing the base of my skull. I close my eyes throughout most of the session. The combination of her warm hands on my scalp, the background music, and the dim light put me in a near comatose state. It would be even better if she were massaging my scalp, but just having someone manipulate and probe your scalp is pretty soothing in its own right. I lose track of time. I am surprised when she turns up the light and announces that the session is complete. Where did the hour go? I tell her how relaxing the session was, and that I normally have a hard time letting go – in line with my Type A personality. My admission of being Type A surprises her, probably because I am wearing my most hippie-appearing clothes, I am unshaven, and I claim to be an author. She comments that when she first was feeling my

CSF pulsations,* they were very frenetic and irregular, but now at the end of the session, they are nice and rhythmic.

I get up slowly. I am very relaxed. I should be hurrying out of the office to pick up Thayer, my youngest son, and take him to his in-line hockey game. Despite my normal Type A-ness, I am too calm to be rushed. First, I must pay the bill. The session costs $75, payable by credit card. I swipe my credit card through a gadget on her cell phone, and in addition to the cost of the visit, I am prompted to add a tip of 15, 20, or 25%. I tip 15%, but am a bit miffed by the request. Am I really supposed to tip someone who owns her own business and who is already pocketing the entire $75 for an hour-long session? Shoot, I never tipped my Rolfer despite spending ten 90-minute sessions with him and developing a pretty close relationship. I understand tipping my waiter or haircutter – and I do so generously – but must I really tip my privately employed massage therapist? My patients don't give me a tip after their infectious disease visits. Is it any different? I am seeking relief from health ailments, and I am already paying a generous amount. I ask my wife about this when I get home, and she confirms that a tip is generally expected in these circumstances. What a strange world we live in.

Despite the awkwardness of the tip, it does little to upset my feeling of calm. I am blissfully relaxed despite coaching my eight-year-old's hockey game that evening. These are some pretty impressive short-term results: remember, I am a tiger dad. I conclude I should have a pretty good next couple of days to weeks now that my CSF rhythms have been

* Cerebrospinal fluid pulsations do appear to be a real phenomenon. I found several studies, mostly involving magnetic resonance imaging (MRI), which confirmed an association between CSF flow and blood flow.[2] I could find no proof that people can actually palpate CSF pulsations. If they can, one would expect the pulsations to roughly correlate with one's blood flow.

restored to normal. I wonder why my CSF rhythm was so irregular to begin with. I give my dad a call. Perhaps he can tell me about the conditions of my undoubtedly traumatic birth, which must have led to my abnormal CSF pulsations. Ideally my mom, the true eyewitness, would have related my birth experience to me, but she passed away four years ago, so my dad will have to do. He is a retired obstetrician and should still be fairly reliable. Contrary to my assumption that my birth was a difficult one, he says it was fast and easy: no nuchal cord around my neck, no need to use forceps to extract me from the birth canal, no extended labor. In fact, I was born on a snowy day in the middle of winter in Minnesota, and my parents actually got in a small fender bender on the way to the hospital. They managed to just make it to the hospital before I popped out. Now my older sister Amy was another story. My mom was in labor a long time with Amy, and the doctor had to use forceps (large metal prongs which grab the infant's head) to help with her delivery. I bet Amy has some really interesting CSF pulsations. Now that I know my delivery was easy, I guess it must be those lifelong hardships that have thrown me out of whack – exactly what those hardships are I am not sure.

A week after the CST session, I assess my general condition. I have a bit of a headache, and my lower back discomfort is unchanged. Reestablishing my CSF rhythm seems to have had no measurable impact. Perhaps I need to go back for another session. Maybe the plumbing of my cerebral system is out of whack again. I did watch the presidential primary debates this week, a traumatic experience or perhaps more of a comedic one. Could that have set me askew once again? No, I think I am done for the time being. After five years, I am ready to reenter the mainstream, maybe not all the way back into mainstream, but I think I am at least done with CST.

As I research the published scientific literature about CST, I come upon several articles regarding the use of CST for Autism Spectrum Disorder (ASD). This is a topic that hits home for me. My oldest son has Asperger's syndrome, recently renamed as high-functioning autism. Due to my obvious skepticism of CST, I am surprised to see the Autism Research Institute, a reputable group, included CST in their list of therapies to treat autism in 2011.[3] CST is also included in a book on *Cutting-edge Therapies for Autism* published in 2010.[4] Wanveer, a certified instructor for the Upledger Institute, was asked by Dr. John Upledger (yes, the very same founding father of modern CST) to address the benefits of CST for Autism. Wanveer hypothesized that persons with autism have increased pro-inflammatory cytokines, neuroglial activation, and inflammatory changes in their cerebral spinal fluid. The inflamed spinal fluid leads to loss of flexibility and likely inflammation of the membrane layers surrounding the brain. These can result in hampering the brain function. He claims that CST is able to "decrease the abnormal and often enormous strain the brain has been under" and thereby help the ASD person "come to newfound levels of tolerance, understanding, and response within themselves and with the world around them."[5]

Once again, I am skeptical. Should my autistic son really receive CST? Connor is a brilliant child. He will want to see proof that CST really works before he gives it a try. I log onto the Autism Research Institute site to confirm they still recommend CST for the treatment of Autism in 2015.[6] What do I find? Nothing. All references to CST have been wiped clean from the site. Apparently, they have had a change of heart. I too am ready to move on.

## Craniosacral Therapy

**Cost:** $60-$125/ hour-long session

**Covered by standard insurance policies:** No

**Published research:** Minimal. A review of the published literature found insufficient evidence to support craniosacral therapy.[7]

# Endnotes


1 Trivieri, L. & Anderson, J.W. *Alternative medicine –the definitive guide* (2nd ed.). Ten Speed Press. 2002.

2 Baledent O, et al. Cerebrospinal fluid dynamics and relation with blood flow: a magnetic resonance study with semiautomated cerebrospinal fluid segmentation. *Invest Radiol,* 2001 Jul;36(7):368-77.

3 Zane, T. A review of craniosacral therapy – science, fads, and applied behavior analysis. *The Current Repertoire*, Fall 2011, Newsletter of the Cambridge Center for Behavioral Studies.

4 Siri, K. & Lyons, T. *Cutting-edge therapies for autism: 2010-2011.* New York, NY: Skyhorse Publishing, 2010.

5 Wanveer, T. Autism spectrum disorder: How craniosacral therapy can help. *Massage Today,* 2007; 7(7), 1-4.

6 http://www.autism.com/ accessed 12/22/2015

7 Green, C., Martin, C.W., Bassett, K., Kazanjian, A. A systematic review of craniosacral therapy: Biological plausibility, assessment reliability and clinical effectiveness. *Complement Ther Med,* 1999 Dec;7(4):201-7.

# Chapter 20 The Final Chapter – Nirvana

I have reached nirvana. According to Buddhism, nirvana is a transcendent state where there is no suffering, desire, or sense of self. I have been going to naturopaths, chiropractors, and their brethren for the past five years. I have certainly reached nirvana by now. Let me take stock: Am I pain-free? Am I healthier? Am I smarter? Am I more relaxed? These are all questions I have been asking myself. We had some family friends over for dinner this past week. The husband is a master woodworker turned orthopedic surgeon, and his wife is a potter when she is not busy mothering their two young children. We were kicking back, drinking some wine when a loud crash, followed by screams, emanated from the basement. The moms sprang into action and reached the scene of the crime before the dads had even registered that something was amiss. When we arrived at the scene, we found our two young boys crawling out from beneath our toppled ping pong table. Their son Joseph had managed to escape the crashing ping pong table. Our seven-year-old son Thayer was not so lucky. He came within a hair of losing an eye. Although a major tragedy had been averted, he still had a big scrape on his face, and a bruise was beginning to form around his eye. The moms took charge while the two doctors were still processing the chain of events. My wife grabbed a bag of frozen peas for Thayer to place on his face. Olive inquired where we kept our arnica. The blank stares with which we answered her question were an answer unto itself. I considered rolling my eyes and saying, “Arnica? Arn’t ya kidding?” but I did not. Remember, I am now educated in the art of alternative medicine, and I am now much more receptive to new ideas, or am I? Olive, suppressing an eye roll of her own, explained that arnica is a homeopathic remedy used to stem bruising and inflammation. (Later, we both realize the use of arnica as Olive described is not homeopathic, but rather a common herbal remedy. Never mind our mistake, it led to an interesting discussion.) She said she always has arnica on hand for incidents such as this.

Once assured that Thayer would survive, we launched into a discussion on the merits of homeopathy. I admitted that of all the alternative therapies I tried, homeopathy ranked near the bottom with regard to my belief that it did any good. I can't stomach the concept that the lower the dose, the more potent the medication, one of the main tenets of homeopathy. The idea that the mere "essence" of the remedy, in the absence of any detectable trace of the named remedy, can have benefit doesn't register as plausible. I could see we were at an impasse in our discussion. Rather than pursue the topic further, we moved on to other subjects. Discussing alternative medicine can be a bit like discussing politics: If you are not in agreement, it doesn't make for polite conversation.

Later that night, while lying down to go to sleep, I thought back to the dinner conversation. Have I not changed over the past five years? Am I still a naysayer when it comes to alternative medicine? I certainly like to say I have changed, but am I being honest with myself? I admit my fallback position when confronted with anything new is skepticism, but no more towards alternative medicine than anything else. Until recently, self-driving cars, Bluetooth, or a Cleveland sports team's winning a championship each seemed quite preposterous, but even these fantasies have become reality.

I argue that I have changed. I am much more willing to consider alternative therapies. Despite my new openness, I also believe alternative medicine is not a panacea. My entire Rolfing experience stemmed from a flare of my lower back pain and my desire for immediate relief. I was desperate for a solution with my trip to Ghana only a week away. Rather than see an internist or orthopedic surgeon, I sought out the assistance of an osteopath and then a Rolfer. Did I recover quickly enough to make my trip to Ghana? No, but my initial visit with the Rolfer led me to follow up and complete the "recipe" of ten recommended Rolfing sessions.

While I don't see myself abandoning Western medicine altogether, I will continue to pick and choose among the alternative therapies that have worked, or at least have shown promise. On the other hand, my practice of infectious diseases will change very little. I understand that the patients who see me expect me to practice traditional evidence-based medicine. What I do for myself is more susceptible to the whims of fancy. When I review my experiences over the past five years, the areas with which I had the most success are hot yoga, pulsed electromagnetic therapy, and sports drinks. The areas from which I derived little benefit, but which I still hold out hope for and may try again, are naturopathic medicine, Ayurveda, barefoot running, detoxification (cleanse), chiropractic care, hypnotism, Rolfing, and acupuncture. By my reckoning, the least beneficial therapies with minimal published evidence are craniosacral therapy, crystal therapy, and homeopathy. Last, there remain some areas of alternative medicine I am not brave enough to try, such as chelation therapy, which involves intravenous administration of agents to bind toxic metal ions. You may also notice there are some areas that I did not include. They were excluded because I ran out of time (five years is long enough) or because they just don't seem radical enough anymore to be called "alternative." Massage, tai-chi, and biofeedback are included in this last category.

There are some common themes that emerged from my experiences. Alternative medicine is more than a single therapy: It is a lifestyle choice. It is hard to sort out what works and what doesn't because the majority of people who embrace alternative medicine are so darn healthy to begin with. The stereotype of the yoga-loving vegan who searches for a connectedness with nature is not too far off base. Proponents of any of the disciplines I investigated will swear to you that the herbs they take or the crystals they wear are the source of their health, but in general, the majority of them live such healthy lifestyles that it is hard to know what to ascribe their well-being to. Don't get me wrong; obese diabetics embrace alternative medicine as well, but probably not as robustly as the barefoot-running vegans.

By and large, my search for scientific validation for the alternative therapies I tried was woefully disappointing. There are few scientifically rigorous studies that have found clear benefit from any of the "alternative" disciplines. There are certainly some small studies that show promise, but by and large, these are trumped by numerous negative studies or no studies at all. Does this mean all alternative therapies are hogwash? Of course not. I certainly benefited from hot yoga, and my athletic performance improved with sports drinks. Even traditional medicine has its warts. Heck, the meniscal repair done on my knee was shown to be no better than a sham surgery in the *New England Journal of Medicine* (the crown jewel of traditional medical publications). I must also admit that some alternative therapies are difficult to study in a rigorous scientific manner. While I recommend keeping an open mind, I do think it pays to research the pros and cons of any treatment. When an HIV-infected patient asks me about whether it is reasonable to rely solely on herbal medicines to treat his HIV disease, I say, "Hell no! You have a disease that will kill you if not treated properly, and I have therapy that is proven – yes, I did say 'proven' – to work." Save the herbs for the non-lethal maladies for which Western medicine does not have good treatment options.

What are some of the pros and cons of Western versus alternative medicine? Pros of Western medicine include: It has evolved over time to reflect our growing knowledge base and our improved understanding of the world. It strives to be evidence based, deriving treatment decisions from randomized, placebo-controlled studies when possible. Due to its evidence-based approach, Western medicine is less reliant on the placebo effect than alternative medicine. Western medicine shines when the placebo effect and spontaneous cure are not enough. Western medicine does have its drawbacks as well. Cons of Western medicine include the following: By virtue of having clear physiological effects, Western medicines not only are beneficial, but may have a higher rate of side effects. Western treatments tend to be more expensive, as anyone who has been unfortunate enough to spend a few days in the hospital is well aware. Last, the Western physician is under increasing time constraints, which often leads to interactions with the patient being shorter and less personal.

What about alternative medicine? Some of the obvious pros of alternative medicine, which I experienced first-hand, include the following: The practitioner typically spends a lot more time with the patient than in Western medicine. This time spent listening to a patient followed by the laying of hands on the patient is an important aspect of the treatment and, correspondingly, patient satisfaction. Alternative medicine relies more heavily on the placebo effect than Western medicine. Homeopathy is a perfect example. Often the prescribed remedy is no more than an inert sugar pill that has been endowed with magical properties. The positive side of this is placebos are less likely to cause serious side effects and can still lead to perceived improvement in a patient's condition, particularly when used for maladies that often resolve on their own, such as viral infection or chronic back pain. I don't mean to discount all alternative therapies as mere placebos. Some alternative therapies have been proven to be effective. Most often when this occurs, the therapy becomes fully adopted by Western medicine or becomes an adjunct to traditional therapy and falls into the category of complementary medicine. Some alternative therapies may have a sound physiologic basis for their benefits, but often this basis is not yet recognized. Alternative medicine tends to be less expensive than Western medicine and generally is very accessible. Drawbacks of alternative medicine often are the flipside of the advantages. Is a placebo effect enough when treating a condition that if unabated may have serious consequences? Should one risk alternative therapy when there is a well-established Western alternative that works, such as anti-viral therapy for HIV infection? Last, even alternative therapies can have toxicities – such as the heavy metals commonly found in Ayurvedic herbal remedies.

I have repeatedly harped on the placebo effect and its large role in alternative medicine and to a lesser extent, Western medicine. What about the placebo effect? Studies have ascribed up to 30% of the benefit from any therapy, alternative or traditional, to the "placebo effect." Basically, if you believe something will help you, there is a reasonable chance it will. When I had my knee surgery, I expected it to work, and as a result, my knee did feel better. Interestingly, after I read the aforementioned *New England Journal of Medicine* article that shed doubt on the benefit of the surgery, my knee started aching again – bye-bye, placebo effect. I no longer believed, and hence some of the perceived benefit was gone. It is also not hard to imagine that some therapies might have a greater placebo effect than others. Acupuncture is a prime example: Having needles stuck into your body from head to toe is a pretty powerful image, and likely ranks high on the "this must be doing something" scale. Alternative practitioners use a lot of gadgets that can seem pretty impressive, such as the traction machine for spinal decompression by the chiropractor and the thumping magnets used for pulsed electromagnetic therapy. These gadgets undoubtedly enhance the placebo effect. While my perception is that most of the alternative practitioners I visited truly believed in the therapy they offered, I could be wrong. Is it ethical to provide a treatment that you know is a sham?

Could the placebo effect be the primary source of benefit from alternative therapies? It is not hard to imagine. If a thousand people try a therapy that has no true benefit, yet 300 of them (30%) perceive a benefit, these same 300 people might openly endorse the therapy, leading to more and more converts. At the same time, the other 700 who had no benefit might try something else rather than openly renounce the therapy. You can see how a vocal minority, composed of the 30% positive responders, could lead to a movement. Is this the basis of alternative medicine's growing appeal?

Perhaps the placebo effect is only part of the answer. Spontaneous cure may also be responsible for some of alternative medicine's successes. There are many conditions which, given time, will resolve on their own. Most viral infections, muscle strains, headaches, and lower back pain come to mind. These are some of the most common conditions for which people seek medical care. Most acute back pain resolves after a few weeks. A few adjustments by the chiropractor over several weeks might be given credit for relief of your pain when, in fact, all you needed was time.

Whatever the reason, be it anecdotes of success, good bedside manner, healthy lifestyles, the placebo effect, or spontaneous cure, one thing is clear: Alternative therapies are here to stay. Even the hospital where I work has gotten into the game, offering acupuncture as part of a new integrative medicine clinic. One of the practitioners in the integrative medicine clinic tells me they are having incredible success in using acupuncture to control pain and decrease the patient's dependence on narcotic pain medicines. At the rate that the public is turning to alternative medicine, we may have to dole out some new labels. Will alternative medicine soon be considered mainstream while Western medicine will be reclassified as "alternative"?

*RAPID LEARNING AND RETENTION THROUGH THE MEDMASTER SERIES:*

**CLINICAL NEUROANATOMY MADE RIDICULOUSLY SIMPLE**, by S. Goldberg
**CLINICAL BIOCHEMISTRY MADE RIDICULOUSLY SIMPLE**, by S. Goldberg
**CLINICAL ANATOMY MADE RIDICULOUSLY SIMPLE**, by S. Goldberg and H. Ouellette
**CLINICAL PHYSIOLOGY MADE RIDICULOUSLY SIMPLE**, by S. Goldberg
**CLINICAL MICROBIOLOGY MADE RIDICULOUSLY SIMPLE**, by M. Gladwin, B. Trattler and C.S. Mahan
**CLINICAL PHARMACOLOGY MADE RIDICULOUSLY SIMPLE**, by J.M. Olson
**OPHTHALMOLOGY MADE RIDICULOUSLY SIMPLE**, by S. Goldberg
**PSYCHIATRY MADE RIDICULOUSLY SIMPLE**, by J. Nelson, W. Good and M. Ascher
**CLINICAL PSYCHOPHARMACOLOGY MADE RIDICULOUSLY SIMPLE**, by J. Preston and J. Johnson
**USMLE STEP 1 MADE RIDICULOUSLY SIMPLE**, by A. Carl
**USMLE STEP 2 MADE RIDICULOUSLY SIMPLE**, by A. Carl
**USMLE STEP 3 MADE RIDICULOUSLY SIMPLE**, by A. Carl
**BEHAVIORAL MEDICINE MADE RIDICULOUSLY SIMPLE**, by F. Seitz and J. Carr
**ACID-BASE, FLUIDS, AND ELECTROLYTES MADE RIDICULOUSLY SIMPLE**, by R. Preston
**THE FOUR-MINUTE NEUROLOGIC EXAM**, by S. Goldberg
**MEDICAL SPANISH MADE RIDICULOUSLY SIMPLE**, by T. Espinoza-Abrams
**CLINICAL ANATOMY AND PHYSIOLOGY FOR THE ANGRY HEALTH PROFESSIONAL**, by J.V. Stewart
**PREPARING FOR MEDICAL PRACTICE MADE RIDICULOUSLY SIMPLE**, by D.M. Lichtstein
**MED'TOONS** (260 humorous medical cartoons by the author) by S. Goldberg
**CLINICAL RADIOLOGY MADE RIDICULOUSLY SIMPLE**, by H. Ouellette and P. Tetreault
**NCLEX-RN MADE RIDICULOUSLY SIMPLE**, by A. Carl
**THE PRACTITIONER'S POCKET PAL: ULTRA RAPID MEDICAL REFERENCE**, by J. Hancock
**ORGANIC CHEMISTRY MADE RIDICULOUSLY SIMPLE**, by G.A. Davis
**CLINICAL CARDIOLOGY MADE RIDICULOUSLY SIMPLE**, by M.A. Chizner
**PSYCHIATRY ROUNDS: PRACTICAL SOLUTIONS TO CLINICAL CHALLENGES**, by N.A. Vaidya and M.A. Taylor.
**PATHOLOGY MADE RIDICULOUSLY SIMPLE**, by A. Zaher
**CLINICAL PATHOPHYSIOLOGY MADE RIDICULOUSLY SIMPLE**, by A. Berkowitz
**ORTHOPEDICS MADE RIDICULOUSLY SIMPLE**, by P. Tétreault and H. Ouellette
**ATLAS OF ORTHOPEDICS**, by P. Tétreault, H. Ouellette, and S. Goldberg
**ANATOMY OF THE SOUL**, by S. Goldberg
**IMMUNOLOGY MADE RIDICULOUSLY SIMPLE**, by M. Mahmoudi
**CLINICAL BIOSTATISTICS MADE RIDICULOUSLY SIMPLE**, by A. Weaver and S. Goldberg

Try your bookstore. For further information, write MedMaster, P.O. Box 640028, Miami FL 33164, or see http://www.medmaster.net. Email: mmbks@aol.com.